Copyright © 2013 Susan Beth Flamm (Puja) RYT

All rights reserved. No part of this publication may be reproduced, stored in a retrieval system, or transmitted in any form or by any means, electronic, mechanical, photocopying, recording or otherwise, without the prior written permission from the author.

Editors: Deborah Klosky and Kalindi E. Trietley
Photographer Pablo Latorre Garcia/Valencia Spain
Book Design: Carie Oltmann
Self published
Second Edition

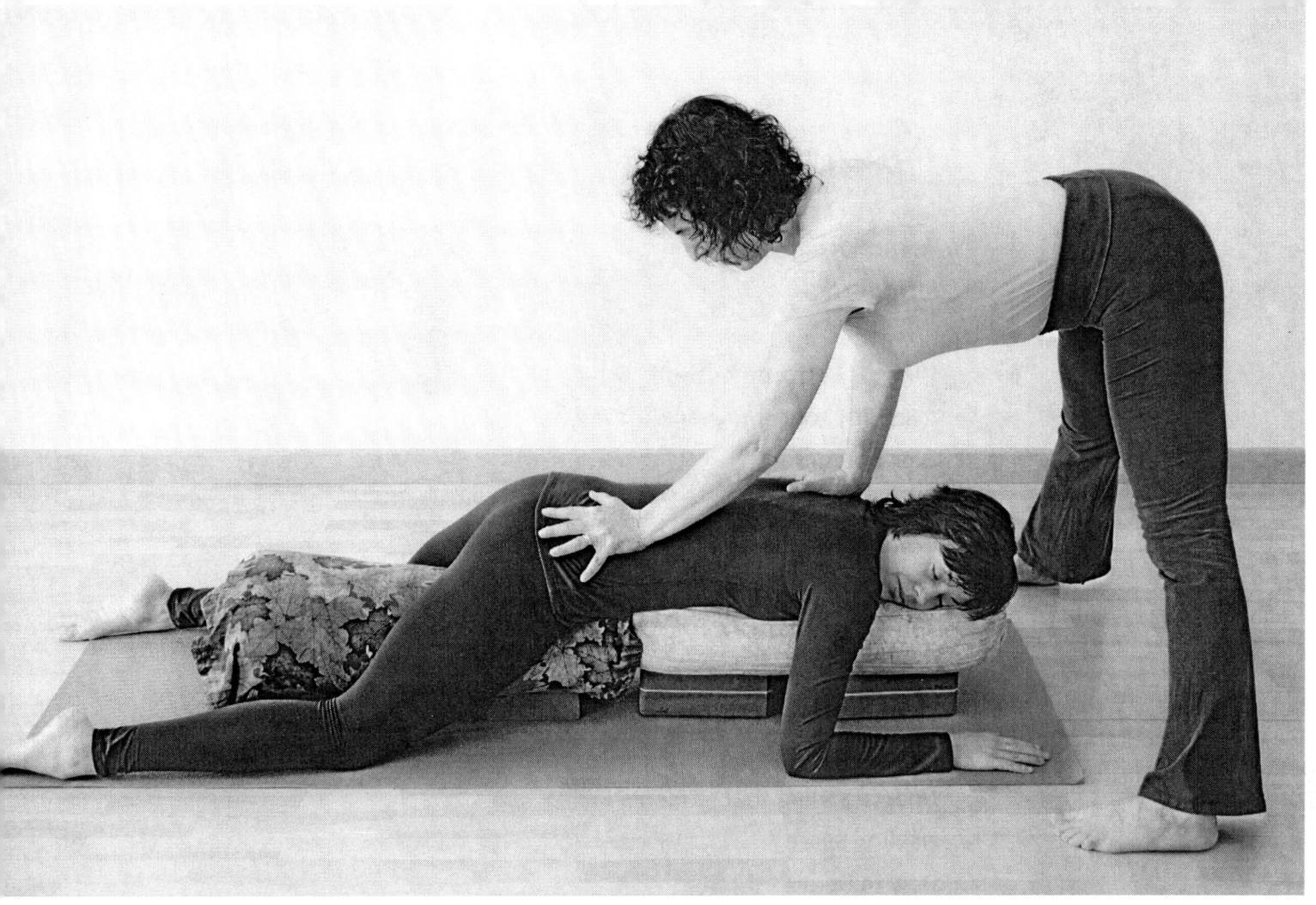

Restorative Yoga with Assists

A Manual for Teachers and Students of Yoga

By Sue Flamm (Puja)

www.pujayoga.net

Contents

Acknowledgments — 9
Introduction — 10

CHAPTER 1 — **What is Restorative Yoga?** — 12
   A Brief History of Yoga in the West — 14
   Explanation — 19

CHAPTER 2 — **What Is The Puja Method of Restorative Yoga?** — 21

CHAPTER 3 — **The Art of Relaxation** — 22

CHAPTER 4 — **Teaching a Restorative Yoga Class** — 24
   Preparing to Teach — 24
   Understanding Your Students — 25
   Holding Space — 26
   How to Demo — 27
   Tone — 27
   Props Needed — 28
   Organization of Students, Props and Space — 30
   Observation and Reading of Students — 30
   Energetics of Alignment — 31

CHAPTER 5 — **Warm-ups to Prepare for Restorative Yoga** — 32
   Creating Your Warm-up Flow — 32

CHAPTER 6 — **Postures and Hands-on Adjustments** — 35
   Touching Students with Consciousness — 35
   Kinds of Touch — 36
   Matching Touch with Students' Needs — 36
   The Energetics of Touch — 37
   How to Protect Your Body and Energy When Assisting Students — 37
   Basic Assists — 38

CHAPTER 7	**Understanding the Nature of The Mind**	**44**
	The Science of the Body, Mind and Stress Connection	44
	Understanding the Nature of the Mind from a Yogic Perspective	47
	Mindfulness	48
	Looking at the Mind from a Quantum Perspective	49
	Mind-Emotion Connection	50
	Staying Out of Your Personal Story	50
	Linking Breath with Thoughts	51
	Affirmations, Mantras and Sounds of the Chakras	51
	Prayer	52
	Gratitude	52
	Visualizations	52
	Calling in Different Energies	54
	Music versus Silence	54
	Helpful Words	55
CHAPTER 8	**Pranayama, Yogic Breath**	**56**
	Full Yogic Breath	56
	Ujjayi Breath	56
	Nadi Shodana	57
CHAPTER 9	**Addressing Different Types of Students**	**58**
CHAPTER 10	**Restorative Asanas (Postures) in Detail**	**60**
	Seated and Forward Bends	**63**
	Supported Baddha Konasana (Supported Cobbler's Pose)	63
	Standing Supported Uttanasana (Standing Supported Forward Bend)	66
	Supported Upavista Konasana (Supported Seated Wide Angle)	68
	Balasana (Supported Child's Pose)	71
	Supported Janu Sirsasana (Seated Angle Head to Knee)	74
	Supported Paschimottanasana (Forward Bend)	76
	Adho Mukha Svanasana (Downward-Facing Dog)	79

Back Bends	**82**
Setubandha Sarvangasana (Supported Bridge)	82
Viparita Dandasana (Backbend with Chair)	86
Inversions	**89**
Viparita Karani (Legs up the Wall)	89
Salamba Sarvangasana (Supported Shoulder Stand)	93
Supine (Lying Down) and Twists	**97**
Supta Baddha Konasana (Reclining Bound Angle Pose)	97
Supta Virasana (Reclining Hero Pose)	103
Supported Supta Padangusthasana (Reclining Big Toe Pose)	107
Utthita Marichyasana (Seated and Standing Twist with Chair)	111
Balasana with Twist (Face Down Forward Reclining Twist with a Bolster)	114
Savasana (Corpse Pose)	117

CHAPTER 11 — *Pregnancy and Beyond: A Special Time in a Women's Life, Getting Pregnant, Prenatal and Postnatal Postures* — **120**

Getting Pregnant	120
Pregnancy	121
Postnatal	122
Restorative Asanas for Pregnancy: Seated and Open Legs, Forward Bends and Elongations	**123**
Supported Baddha Konasana (Supported Cobbler's Pose)	123
Standing Supported Uttanasana (Standing Supported Forward Bend, Open Legs)	126
Supported Upavista Konasana (Supported Seated Wide Angle)	128
Balasana (Supported Child's Pose)	131
Supported Janu Sirsasana (Seated Angle Head to Knee)	134
Adho Mukha Svanasana (Downward-Facing Dog)	137
Pregnancy Inversions	**140**
Salamba Sarvangasana (Supported Shoulder Stand)	140
Pregnancy Supine (Lying Back) and Side Lying	**143**
Supta Baddha Konasana (Reclining Bound Angle Pose)	143
Supta Virasana (Reclining Hero Pose)	148
Savasana (Corpse Pose)	151

CHAPTER 12	***Sequencing for Your Class or Individual Students***	**154**
	Working with Specific Conditions	154
	Sequences: Getting Pregnant, Pre-Pregnancy	155
	Pregnancy	156
	Postnatal 1	157
	Postnatal 2	158
	Stress, Anxiety, Fibromyalgia, Chronic Fatigue	159
	Depression (long)	161
	Depression (short)	162
	Depression (shorter)	163
	Exhaustion	164
	Headache	165
	PMS	166
	Menstruation	168
	Menopause	171
	About the Author and Models	**174**
	References	**176**

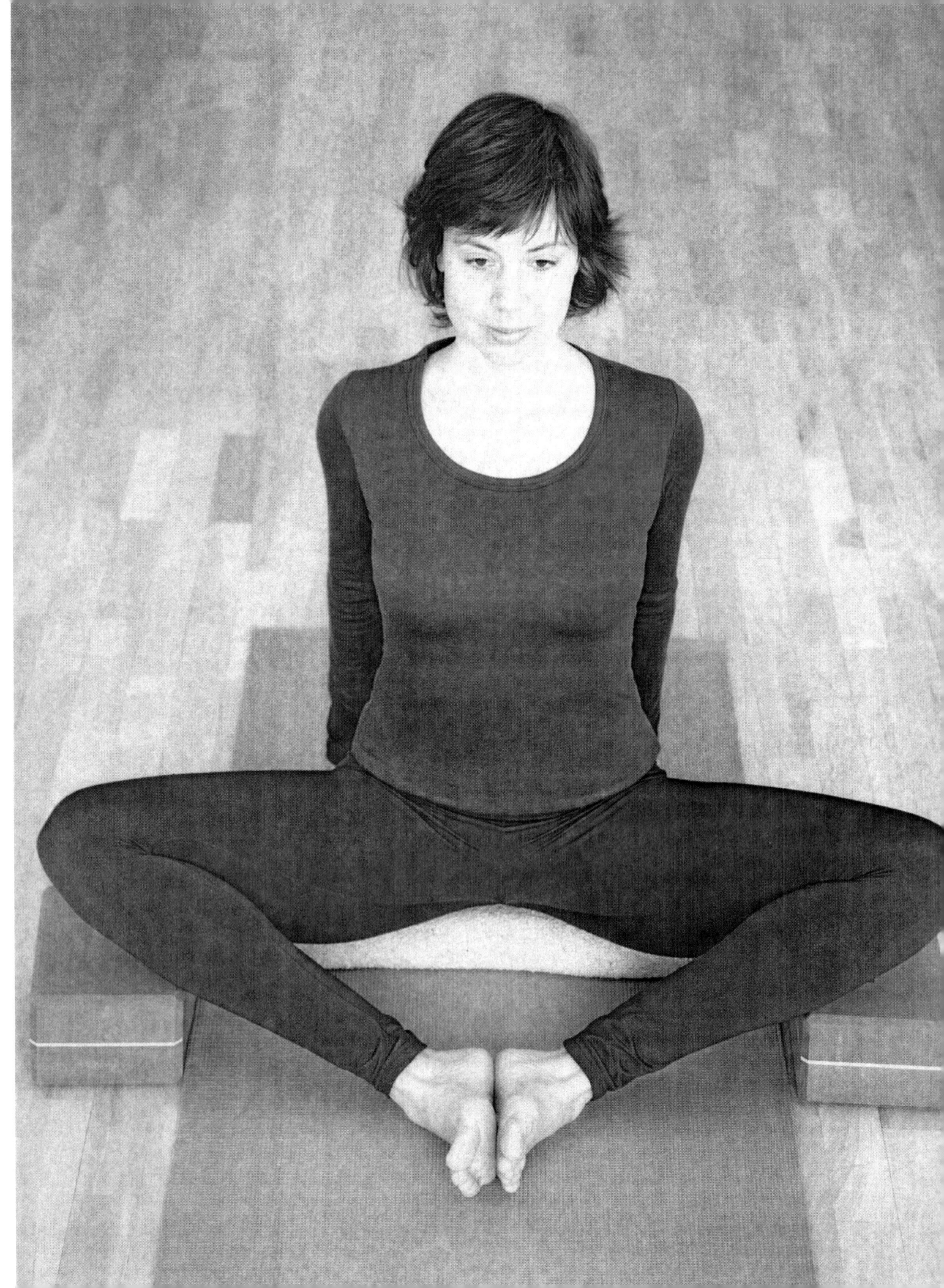

Acknowledgments

I would like to acknowledge the following people for their support of me and of this book: First, my dear husband René for his continual love, encouragement from the beginning to the end of this project and his ideas to make this book even better. My sweet and beautiful twelve-year-old daughter Elena who helped me with spelling and editing and for her support and patience waiting to use the computer while I was busy writing and researching. My editor, Debbie Klosky, for her positive attitude, support and invaluable help with the editing process. Carmela Escriche Mengual for her support and generosity in using her elegant studio for the photo shoots. Pablo Latorre Garcia for his excellent photographic skills, patience and attention to detail. Ella, for her attention to detail in the photo shoots and, with Alma, for their loving support during the photo shoots. Jenny Susan Kaiser and Julia, my amazing models who gave their time and wonderful energies for the photos. Mabel for her assistance in hair and makeup for the photo shoot. Arti Ross Kelso for her continual support, friendship and time with editing the bodywork chapter of the book. Susan Rubin for her encouragement, ideas, editing and continual support for my teaching and especially my Restorative Teacher Training. Kalindi for her editing and general support for the project. Carie Oltmann for her genorousity and expertise in design. Eileen Muir for introducing me to restorative yoga and for her wonderful work in the yoga world. My mom for always, always supporting me in everything. And all of my students, teachers and fellow seekers on the yogic path who have each in their own way been the inspiration for the creation of this book.

Introduction

My life has been a continual journey of learning, self-discovery and service. I took my first Transcendental Meditation course at 12 years of age, and my first Hatha Yoga class at 16. They both felt somehow familiar to me and laid a foundation for my journey with yoga, so with many steps along the path of yoga, I've felt taken back home to my essential self.

About 28 years ago, my practice deepened significantly as I began to walk on "the path of love" with Kripalu Yoga. I chose to live at that Center for six years to immerse myself in the yogic lifestyle. After that, I studied a variety of different yoga styles – Iyengar, Ashtanga (Mysore style), and Anusara – all with wonderful instructors. I directed and owned two yoga studios with all levels of classes including ongoing restorative classes.

In my second studio in Amherst, MA, USA (about 15 years ago), my business partner and I invited a number of teachers to give intensive workshops there. One of those teachers was Judith Lasater. She had just completed her book, *Rest and Renew*. Although I had practiced and taught restorative yoga before, I had never experienced anyone with Judith's mastery. I became absorbed deeply in her methods of instruction, especially during those times when she took my hand and pointed out nuances with student after student. What a wonderful experience. From that time on, restorative yoga has become an integral part of my yoga practice and teaching.

It seems to me that the potential of this special line of yoga is far reaching. I have had the opportunity to patiently and lovingly guide a wide variety of students, and I've seen some amazing things. One woman who had been my student for several years became seriously ill with a rare form of cancer. She asked me to work with her privately. Unfortunately there were not very many private sessions, because she soon left this world. During that time though, I "held the space" for her while she rested in restorative poses, and her process was an absolute gift for me. She taught me about relaxing not only into life, but also into death (another significant deepening for me).

I have also worked with students recovering from serious illness, students with a variety of disabilities, and students who are simply stressed out. Each one had a particular need and a particular gift to give. Each seems to have opened and changed to one degree or another. I think most yoga teachers discover this dynamic.

Over time, I found that I wanted to share all I had learned with other teachers. I began to focus on the art of teaching in various teacher-oriented workshops and training sessions, but still I felt the desire to create something more in-depth, more comprehensive – something that included both the heart and the intricacies of this unique style of yoga. Now I'm ready to take the next step with this book. I have integrated much of my learning from bodywork and years of yogic practice into a restorative yoga practice that I have come to call the Puja Method, or as it has sometimes been referred to, Puja Yoga.

There is a part of this book that is not written, which is the ongoing, constantly changing internal perception and experience of the practitioner in the restorative asanas. I use as a tool to encourage my students these four steps in which to be with the pose:

Enter: Enter inside of your body.
Perceive and investigate: Become perceptive to what is happening inside and investigate.
Accept: Accept your current state with compassion and loving kindness.
Relax: Relax around all that you feel on the physical level, all that you have perceived in your body, mind, emotions and on any other level of your being.

I invite you to use these steps with your students and with your own exploration of this beautiful and transformative practice.
Before I go on, I want to say that it has been an absolute honor to work with so many students and teachers throughout the years, and to share the life journey that yoga provides. I hope some of you will enjoy seeing my progress. May you all receive many blessings in your teaching, exploration and practice.

A note on references: I refer to different books and websites throughout the book. The reader can find the complete references used for each chapter collected at the end of the book.

CHAPTER 1

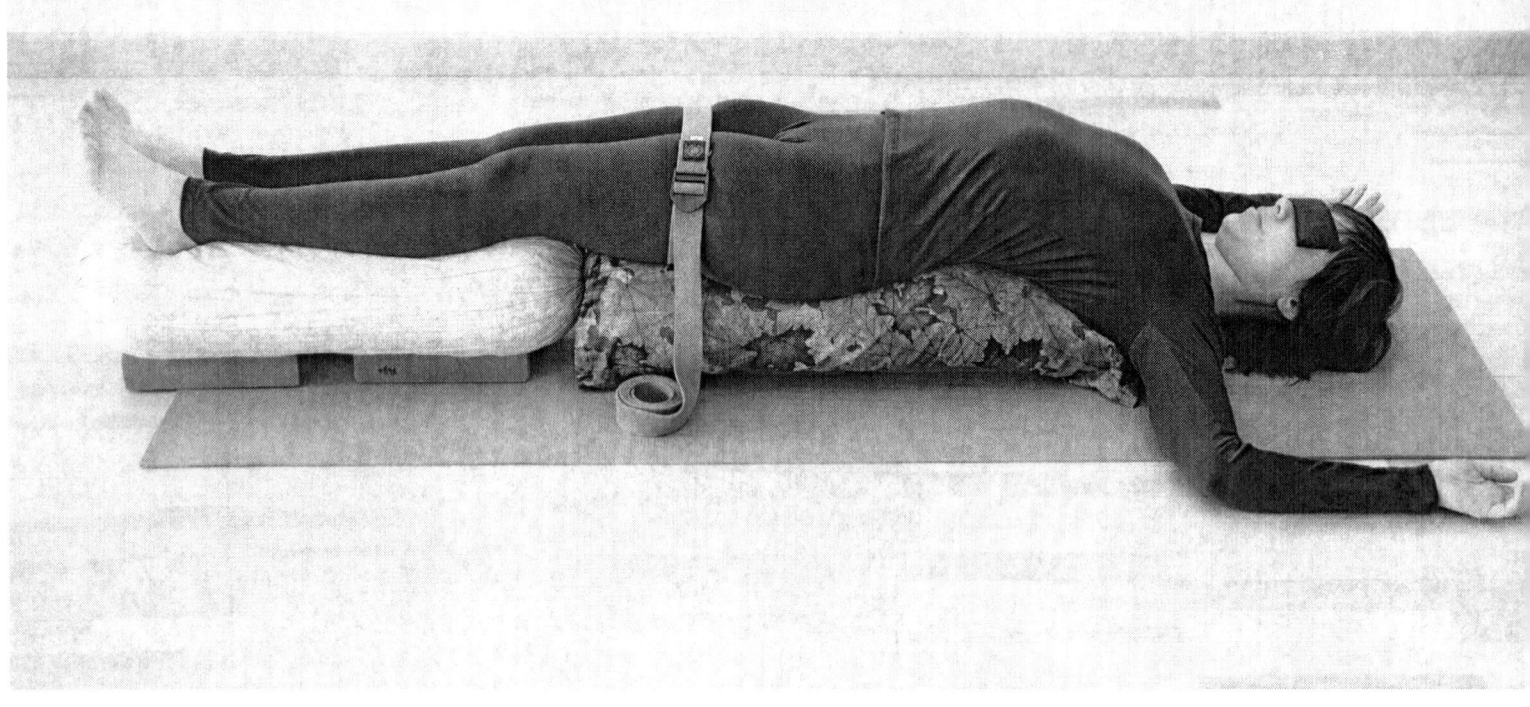

What is "Restorative Yoga"?

"Never perform asanas mechanically."
B.K.S. Iyengar

I would like to give you both a very small overview of yoga in general and where "Restorative Yoga" fits into that world. Yoga, as a more than 5,000-year-old tradition, has a history that is vast and ancient.

Patanjali, who is described as a writer, physician, philosopher and saint, is considered by many to be the grandfather of yoga. His Yoga Sutras, originally written in Sanskrit, are one of the most widely respected texts on yoga. There is some controversy over exactly when they were written, though 200 BC is quoted in many texts.

The Yoga Sutras are a series of 196 sutras or aphorisms about yoga and have been translated and interpreted by many. The first four are:

"This is the teaching of yoga. (1)
Yoga is the cessation of the turnings of thought. (2)
When thought ceases, the spirit stands in its true identity as observer to the world. (3)
Otherwise the observer identifies with the turning of thought. (4)

The first four aphorisms of Patanjali define the nature of yoga as a state of mental tranquility and spiritual freedom, as well as the means to achieve this state."
Yoga: Discipline of Freedom: The Yoga Sutras Attributed to Patanjali, translated by Barbara Stoler Miller

Yoga as defined by B.K.S. Iyengar: *"The word Yoga is derived from the Sanskrit root yuj meaning to bind, join, attach and yoke, to direct and concentrate one's attention on, to use and apply. It also means union or communion. It is the true union of our will with the will of God."* Light on Yoga

When the word "God" is used I equate that word with love or the higher self. Yoga is not a religion, it is a science and for some a lifelong practice. These definitions touch on the study and practice of yoga, which is multilayered and multifaceted. To understand and master any art, much study and practice is required. One does not become a black belt or understand what it means to be a black belt the moment the student enters the dojo, nor does one become a master bricklayer by building a brick wall or a doctor by putting on scrubs and listening to someone's heartbeat with a stethoscope. These are things that must be studied, practiced and understood. As in yoga, this is a lifelong study that continues to reveal itself with years of practice and dedication. Yoga is not perfecting positions, or yoga asanas, it is so much more. Yoga is a living practice. What is revealed to us on the yoga mat serves as a metaphor for our lives. The more outwardly focused our world becomes the more popularity yoga gains as a means of balancing a very out-of-balance reality that we have created here on planet Earth.

The original yoga practice is still being followed by many. At the same time there are many teachers and practitioners who still have much to learn about this time-honored art. There are yoga teacher training certifications that are a weekend course. This is a disservice to this precious and profound body of knowledge and art.

A Brief History of Yoga in the West

Yoga came to the west in stages. Here is a timeline of when some of the major lineages or traditions of yoga came to the United States and Canada:

1893	Yoga and its teachings with its long history first comes to the United States through a visit to Chicago by India's Swami Vivekenanda.
1920	Paramahansa Yogananda establishes the Self Realization Fellowship in the United States. His teachings are now also taught under the name of *Ananda Yoga* and the *Self Realization Fellowship*.
1959	Swami Vishnudevananda, founder of Sivananda Yoga, opens a center in Montreal.
1960	Amrit Desai comes to the United States, after years of teaching yoga; in 1972 he founds *Kripalu Yoga Ashram*.
1960's	Maharishi Mahesh Yogi's *Transcendental Meditation* gains popularity in the West.
1966	Swami Satchidananda, founder of *Integral Yoga*, arrives in New York City.
1967	B.K.S. Iyengar publishes *Light on Yoga*.
1969	Yogi Bhajan brings *Kundalini Yoga* to the United States.
1969	Swami Rama comes to the United States and founds the *Himalayan Institute*.
1970	Bikram Choundry, founder of *Bikram Yoga*, opens the first Yoga College of India in Hawaii.
1970's	Lilias Folan hosts the *Yoga and You* series on PBS.
1971	Swami Muktananda brings *Siddha Yoga* to the United States.
1973	B.K.S. Iyengar comes to teach in Ann Arbor, Michigan.
1975	Pattabhi Jois visits the United States and introduces *Ashtanga Yoga*.
1975	*Yoga Journal* magazine is founded in San Francisco.
1976	T.K.V. Desikachar visits the United States.

Adapted from Cynthia Worby, *The Everything Yoga Book* pp.27, 28

Since then, from the 80s and 90s to today, 50 plus styles of yoga have been formed and founded by Americans, Australians and Europeans; a few examples of these are: Jivamukti Yoga, David Life and Sharon Gannon; Yoga Zone, Alan Finger; Anusara Yoga, John Friend; Viniyoga, Gary Kraftsow; Tri Yoga, Kali Ray; Forrest Yoga, Ana Forrest; and many more.

Many of these teachers studied one or more of the previously mentioned main schools of yoga with one of these Indian teachers or gurus who came to the West; some also journeyed to India to study with their gurus. There are now offshoots and interpretations, variations and combinations, that also exist and keep being created.

There are many approaches to this ancient tradition. Just as there are many paths to reach the top of a mountain and many roads that will take you to the same place, there are several prominent paths from the Indian yogic tradition of yoga; for our purposes I will focus briefly on the following three: Raja Yoga, Karma Yoga and Bhakti Yoga. Each of these paths has a distinct focus but all have the same end union--yoga, communion with the highest within you, communion with love, union with all that is.

I have included these three because I feel they all relate to the practice and teaching of restorative yoga. The practice of yoga is not only a physical practice. It is much more. Working with, understanding and quieting the mind is integral in the knowledge and practice of yoga.

Raja Yoga

Raja Yoga is often referred to as the royal path for this reason. Within each of us lives witness consciousness, mindfulness, a higher self, a wise queen or king that can think clearly, make clear decisions and is not swayed by the ideas or ramblings of others who may be reflecting a lack of clarity inside their own mind. Raja Yoga is also called Ashtanga Yoga, the eight (ashta) limbs (anga) that the system rests on.

"Ashtanga - The Eight Limbs of Raja Yoga
Often called the 'royal road,' it offers a comprehensive method for controlling the waves of thought by turning our mental and physical energy into spiritual energy. Raja Yoga or Ashtanga Yoga referring to the eight limbs leading to enlightenment. When body and energy are under control meditation comes compiled by the Sage Patanjali Maharishi in the Yoga Sutras, the Eight Limbs are a series of disciplines which purify the body and mind, ultimately leading the yogi to enlightenment."
http://www.self-realization.com/articles/yoga/yoga_systems.htm

"He who has conquered his mind is a Raja Yogi. The word Raja means king."
Light on Yoga, p. 22

These 8 limbs are:

1. **Yamas** - The Yamas or restraints (Don'ts) are divided into five parts. They can be practiced in thought, speech and action.
    a. Ahimsa - non-violence.
    b. Satya - truthfulness, speaking and living truthfully.
    c. Brahmacharya - moderation in all things (control of all senses). Practicing integrity in intimate and sexual relationships.
    d. Asteya - non-stealing, not taking something from another that is not yours.
    e. Aparigraha - non-wishing for what someone else has.
2. **Niyamas** - The Niyamas or observances (Do's) are also divided into five parts:
    a. Saucha or purity - referring to internal thoughts and to the physical body, internal and external cleanliness.
    b. Santosha - contentment; with what is and what isn't.
    c. Tapas - austerity, living simply, dropping the desire for more.
    d. Swadhyaya - study of the sacred texts, spirituality and wisdom.
    e. Ishwara Pranidhana - to live with an awareness of the divine presence and that you are a part of that.

This idea that we are a part of everything and connected to all of existence here on the earth is reflected in this quote: *"The earth does not belong to man, man belongs to the earth. All things are connected like the blood that unites us all. Man did not weave the web of life, he is merely a strand in it. Whatever he does to the web, he does to himself."* From a speech by Chief Seattle of the Duwamish Native American tribe

3. **Asana** - yoga postures.
4. **Pranayama** - regulation or breath control.
5. **Pratyahara** - withdrawal of the senses.
6. **Dharana** - concentration
7. **Dhyana** - meditation
8. **Samadhi** - the superconscious state. In Samadhi non-duality or oneness is experienced.

In regards to the yamas and niyamas, Bapuji Swami Kripaluvanandaji said when you take one bead from the mala to pick it up, all the other beads come with it. It is the same with the practice of the yamas and niyamas--practice one and all the others will follow naturally.

These eight limbs are not necessarily to be practiced or taught in order, perfecting each one, but they all can be integrated within the practice at the same or different moments.

Restorative yoga as a part of Raja Yoga or Ashtanga Yoga, the eight limbs of yoga, connects to a part of the third limb, asana, but includes all the other limbs of the Ashtanga practice as well. The 1st and 2nd limbs, yamas and niyamas, deal more with attitude and the approach to working with the body and mind; the 4th limb is pranayama, yogic breath; the 5th pratyahara, the withdrawal of the senses; the 6th dharana, concentration; the 7th dhyana, meditation; and the 8th is entering to moments of pure connection and contentment. All of these limbs can be experienced through the restorative practice.

Karma Yoga

Karma Yoga is the yoga of action or selfless service. I practiced this form of yoga with great intensity for six years while living at Kripalu Yoga Center for Yoga and Health in Lenox, MA, in the USA, when it was both an ashram, teaching and learning center. Karma Yoga continues to be an integral part of my practice. We worked six-and-a-half days a week and we offered all our work in the service of the highest. That is to say, we offered our work in the service of all the guests who came to practice and learn yoga and healing arts, to our fellow seekers on the path and to our teachers who taught us the yogic practices and ways. We were dedicated and worked from our hearts. We made $35 a month and had all our food and shelter taken care of. We worked as an act of service to humanity. It was one of the most beautiful times in my life.

I still consider my teaching service, and though it is my way of earning a living, few get wealthy being a yoga teacher. I feel so blessed to have the opportunity to be in the presence of personal transformation on every level that I have had the honor to witness in my students as they continue to practice and understand the meaning of yoga, and as I see their practice reflected in their lives.

"Karma Yoga is the Yoga of Action. It is the path chosen primarily by those of an outgoing nature. It purifies the heart by teaching you to act selflessly, without thought of gain or reward. By detaching yourself from the fruits of your actions and offering them up to God, you learn to sublimate the ego. To achieve this, it is helpful to keep your mind focused by repeating a mantra while engaged in any activity."
http://www.sivananda.org/teachings/fourpaths.html#jnana

As a teacher of restorative yoga, Karma Yoga comes into play with the attitude that your teaching is a service. You are serving your students and the planet by teaching and assisting your students to connect with themselves more deeply. You are assisting your students in understanding what it means to relax and facilitating healing through the practice.

"Karma Yoga is the selfless devotion of all inner as well as the outer activities as a Sacrifice to the Lord of all works, offered to the eternal as Master of all the soul's energies and austerities." - Bhagavad Gita

Bhakti Yoga

Bhakti Yoga is the path of devotion or divine love. I also practiced this while living at Kripalu Center and beyond. My spiritual name given to me while living at Kripalu, Puja, is a yogic ceremony of offering the five elements —earth, water, fire, air and ether— to a deity or the highest in any living being. A deity is a representation of a divine aspect or aspects that we all have with in us. So when we perform a puja ceremony, for example, we are honoring that aspect of our being and cultivating those characteristics in our own being. Other forms of Bhakti Yoga are prayer and chanting, along with other ceremonies and rituals.

Similarly, I consider the practice of Bhakti Yoga to be an integral part of the restorative practice. I look to see the divinity in each of my students. I teach to that place and cultivate that place within each of them. I consider it an absolute honor to be a yoga teacher and to be able to be witness the transformation I see happening in my students.
B.K.S. Iyengar is the founder of restorative yoga with props. He has been teaching and practicing yoga for more than 75 years, and is the author of 19 yoga books in-

cluding the yoga bible, *Light on Yoga*, and *YOGA, The Path to Holistic Health*, which includes wonderful asana sequences, with both traditional and restorative asanas, for a variety of physical, mental and emotional conditions. Through his ingenuity and experience working with many students, he developed a system of using props to make yoga available to everyone no matter their age or physical condition. His use of props also allows students to go deeper into the asanas and be supported in their practice. I believe that Iyengar would say all yoga is "restorative" but this particular approach of using props to support the relaxation and deepening process has taken on this name within the Iyengar tradition. I have also seen other "styles" call certain sequences or poses "restorative" but with this term I am addressing a particular approach and techniques that I first experienced in Iyengar yoga as developed by B.K.S. Iyengar as well as my own approach to this very special practice.

Judith Lasater, a world-renowned, dedicated yoga teacher, physical therapist and Ph.D, expanded this unique approach in the West through both her teachings and her invaluable book, *Relax and Renew*. There is no doubt that she has had and continues to have a deep impact on the yogic community for students and teachers alike. She has exposed many practitioners to a fuller experience of the restorative practice of yoga. I am fortunate to have been one of those students.

Explanation

Today some yoga styles use restorative poses as part of their practice to address different conditions and needs of students. Restorative yoga as I refer to it in this book is not a new style or school of yoga, it is a selection of poses, many that include props to help the practitioner explore deep relaxation, stillness, inner peace and many physical benefits of the yoga practice. Restorative yoga as I teach it combines supported postures (asanas) with conscious breath (pranayama), relaxation and techniques to still and calm the body and mind.

Restorative yoga explores the capacity of individual students to relax deeply, to understand their bodies and minds more intimately, and to open their hearts more fully to love. Generally speaking, in the restorative practice we move through a progressive series of postures using various props for support. When the body is supported by these props—blankets, bolsters, blocks, straps, eye bags, walls and chairs—the body, mind and spirit are given the message to let go of deeply held tension. We end the session with the most basic restorative asana—savasana (corpse pose).

Each pose has a variety of benefits, which I will discuss in some detail as we continue. With each posture, however, students learn the "art of relaxation," which brings them into a place of peace and tranquility. When deep relaxation is realized, healing can happen on many levels. This unique approach allows for an exploration of the very essence of yoga—union.

CHAPTER 2

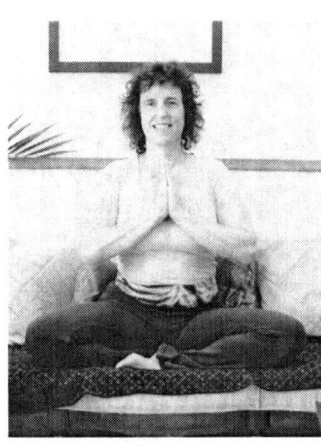

What Is The Puja Method of Restorative Yoga?

After almost 40 years of practicing yoga and meditation, and 30 years of teaching them, I have now developed my own method of restorative yoga, which I call the Puja Method of Restorative Yoga. It is a synthesis of what I've learned from many extraordinary teachers, my personal practice and from my own body and mind explorations.

"Where there is love there is life"
Mahatma Ghandi

The principles of the Puja Method are:
- Cultivating compassion and loving kindness through your words, thoughts and actions as a teacher or practitioner.
- Working to cultivate a deeper understanding of the mind and using techniques to calm and quiet the mind.
- Understanding and applying hands-on assists to traditional restorative yoga asanas.
- Understanding and facilitating deep relaxation through various techniques including asana, pranayama, visualization, meditation, stillness, breath, and hands-on assists.

The intention is for teachers and students to embrace this integrated system so they can be even more responsive to their students and to themselves. As they come to understand not only body alignment and how to individualize adjustments for each student's particular physical needs, but also the interface among body, mind, emotions and spirit, a more powerful experience of healing is allowed to happen.

CHAPTER 3

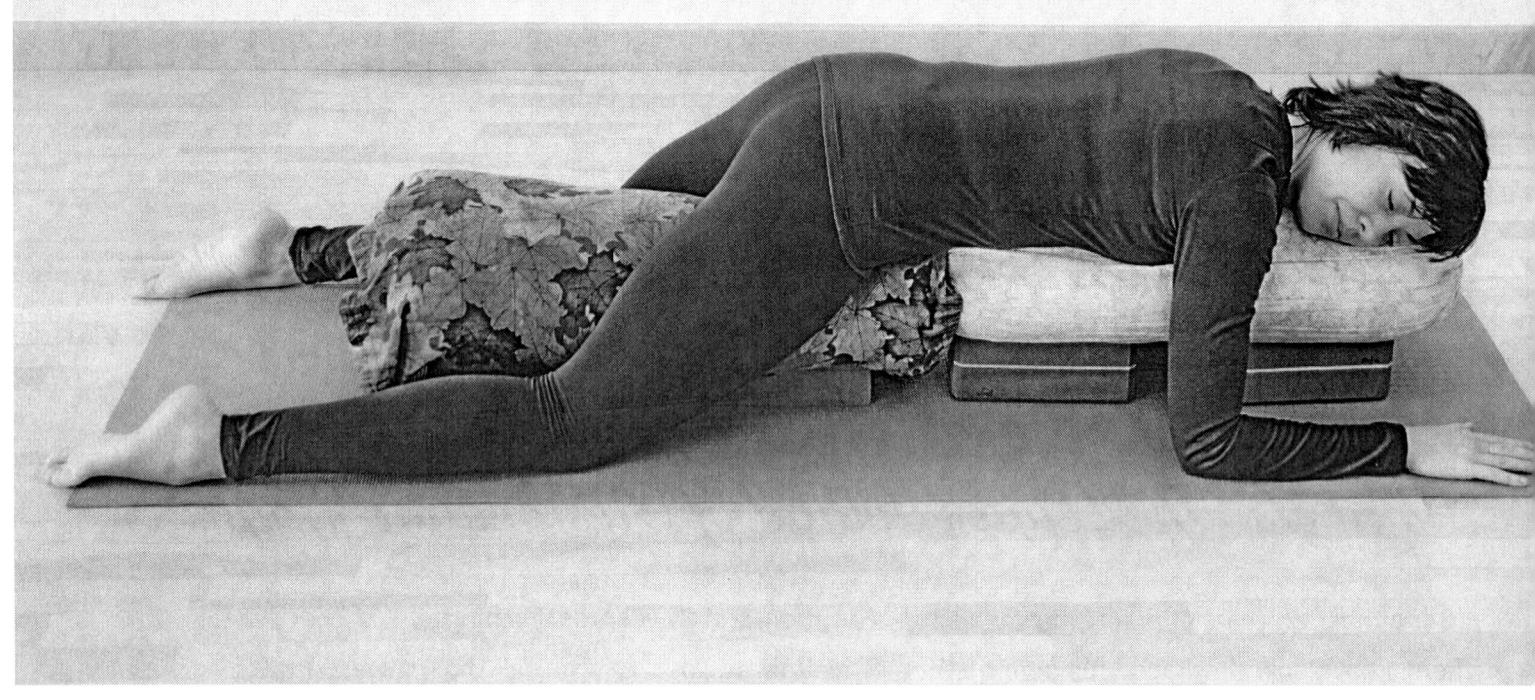

The Art of Relaxation

"Take rest; a field that has rested gives a bountiful crop." Ovid (Publius Ovidius Naso)

Living in these challenging times, we all experience stress at a number of different levels. Most of us are not even aware how deep the effects of stress can go. There can be real repercussions when stress is unrecognized and unaddressed. Acute and degenerative diseases of the body and mind have been linked directly to unresolved tension.

Relaxation has become foreign to many, but its benefits are truly far reaching. There have been countless studies on the effects of relaxation on illness and general lack of well being. Here are a few of the benefits of deep relaxation and restorative yoga:

- Promotes inner peace and tranquility
- Improves memory
- Increases concentration
- Increases mental clarity
- Supports immune system function
- Soothes the nervous system
- Releases stress
- Improves circulation to and function of organs and organ systems
- Alleviates discomforts associated with menstruation, pregnancy and menopause
- Regulates blood pressure
- Reduces or eliminates depression
- Reduces or eliminates dependency on medications
- Relieves or reduces headaches
- Supports the recovery from illness

There have been many studies on the effects of relaxation that have documented and confirmed the many benefits of the ability to create relaxation in the body. There are several techniques and levels of relaxation. Many of us walk around with unconscious stress in our shoulders, belly, back or other part of the body, not aware of the degree to which these areas are tense. Most of us cannot complete our daily to-do's each day and are often overburdened with responsibilities of family, work and life. We are all trying to find a balance but our scales are often tipped to the stress side.

The ability to facilitate relaxation and to be able to relax in yourself is an art that must be practiced like anything you want to become proficient at. Some of us are more easygoing than others, but stress is inherent to being human. We are continually cultivating ways to reduce stress and move repeatedly into a more peaceful and relaxed place so we can meet everything which comes to us in our lives with more compassion, kindness and clarity.

Learning the art of relaxation is like working a muscle. We can relax more easily when we have paved the way for the relaxation to enter. Restorative Yoga and working with the mind through the techniques offered in this book will give you the tools you need to both facilitate relaxation in others and cultivate relaxation in yourself.

CHAPTER 4

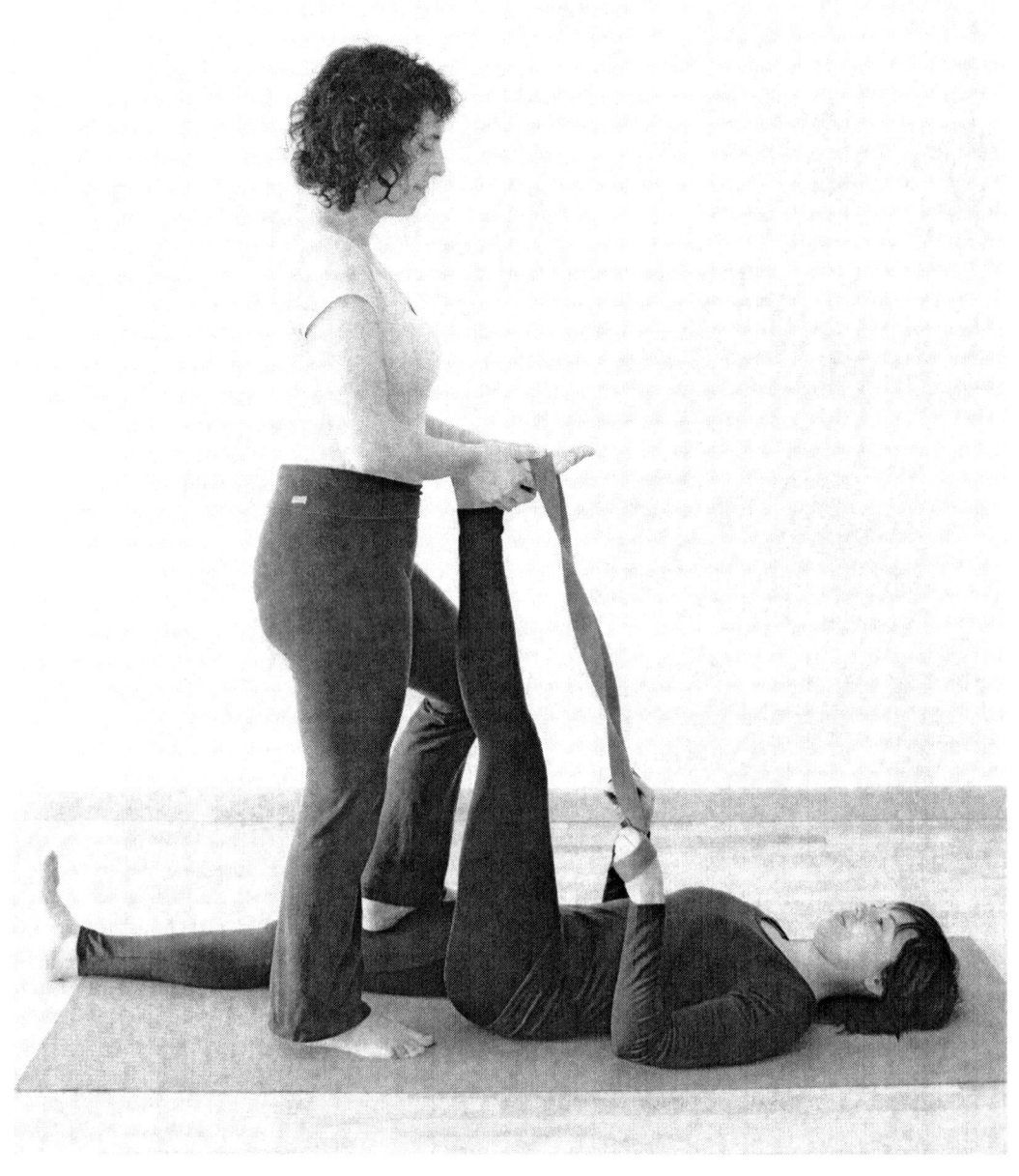

Teaching a Restorative Yoga Class

Preparing to Teach

"Smile, breathe, and go slowly."
Thich Nhat Hanh

When you prepare for your restorative yoga class, you might like to create a ritual for yourself. That can be a simple prayer of asking to be open to guidance, a brief meditation, or some centering and calming breath. Of course you also want to make detailed plans, like sequences, specific techniques, desirable props, etc. Still, the details won't work nearly as well without attention to the deeper aspects of the yogic practice.

Remember you are teaching to serve your students. Teach to what they are needing. If you know who your students are prepare to teach to what will support them. If you don't know them consider using this opportunity to get to know them. It is important to remember that as a teacher, you are a conduit of energy in your classes. Energy flows from you to your students. Your voice, your touch, your energy is being felt by your students, each one of them at some level. We are vibrational beings, and your students will pick up on your vibration as a teacher and begin to resonate with your energy. You can easily understand why it's wise to take some responsibility for your energy state before beginning to teach.

Allow yourself to feel prepared for your class, so you can feel relaxed and fully present. Look inside to know what that means for you. You might want to write out a sequence (or more than one); you might want to have an inspirational reading selected. No matter how good your plan, however, you have to be willing to make adjustments as needed. This will become easier as you get to know your students. Even then, you must look at your students with fresh eyes in every class. That intention is a good part of every plan.

Understanding Your Students

When we teach a yoga class, we develop a relationship with each student, and we also help to create a class energy. At the beginning of each class, take time to check in with your students either individually or in a group. Try to arrive 15 minutes early to greet your students as they come in. If there isn't time to check in with each one individually, ask the class about their state of mind and body once they are all seated. You might open with: "Is there anything of particular interest or concern going on with anyone?"

When there are new students, make a special point to connect with them and find out about why they have come. Walk over and introduce yourself; speak personally and with compassionate attention. Ask specifically about their physical and mental situation.

When you have all this updated information about your students, you may want to tailor your class to address one or more of the concerns that have been mentioned. Sometimes you will find themes with your students; for instance, four of your students may have neck issues. If you've spent a little time before class anticipating some of the most frequent issues, you'll only need a moment during class to think about how you want to continue. For instance, if you've created and practiced several different flows, shifting from one to the other is not difficult at all.

When I sit in front of a group, several dynamics come into play. I may have planned something to teach, but I may receive guidance from either my students' sharing, or from my intuition. I am always willing to drop my plan for that day's class and adjust to address the needs of my students. When you begin to understand your students, you develop the ability to read them. As your experience grows, you can trust increasingly in your abilities as a teacher to make last-minute changes in your design. If this is challenging for you it is okay to stick to your original plan too, especially in the beginning.

It is always good to come with a plan; just be willing to toss it out if it doesn't address the needs of your students.

Holding Space

What does it mean to "hold space"? It might mean creating a physical space that includes candles, an altar, or soft music; but what is more important is that it means bringing your presence to be in the moment with your students. Bring yourself into a receptive, loving, empty place inside; and that helps you enter into the moment with your students. It's the greatest gift you can give them. From that centered place, you are not thinking about what you are going to make for dinner that night, or your personal problems. Instead you are maintaining a meditative space in which your students can deepen in their practice. They can feel held in compassion and presence.

How do you bring yourself into a receptive, loving and empty place inside? Put all of your personal worries and concerns to the side. For the time that you will be teaching, if you have a problem letting go of your personal problems give them over to the spirit, a god or goddess, a higher power, your angels or whoever you relate to so that during class you are available to be receptive to your students' needs. Come early into class and meditate, enter into prayer, chant or do some yoga to bring you into your center. When you are in your center you are able to be more connected to those around you.

How to Demo

Restorative practice uses props that require special attention when instructing your students. When you are ready to begin a new pose:
Set up your props first.
Then have your students get their props and set them up.
When everyone has their props ready, invite them to come gather around so each student can see and hear the instructions.
Begin by explaining and demonstrating the pose yourself, or use a student as a model. (When using a student ask permission and always thank them after they have finished.)

When you have a class that knows the postures, and you want to integrate someone new, have your students that know how to get into the pose do so, and then you assist the new students as needed. Use the students that know the pose as models for the one who is just learning. Always be aware of the individual needs of your students, if possible, and demonstrate any variations that may be necessary. It's good to mention variations more often when you have a newer class, or some new members. Taking these simple steps will allow your class to flow more smoothly, and that's what we are looking for – smooth flows as we teach.

Tone

Be aware of your voice. Speak clearly and softly, but loudly enough for all to hear. Your voice is one medium for transmitting an energy vibration for your students to connect with, so allow your voice to carry the energy of your compassionate and loving heart. That doesn't mean sounding like you're in a trance, though, nor does it mean forcing people to strain to catch your words. Consider the proper balance, especially if you have older students in the room, a large class or poor acoustics.

Props Needed

Depending on the particular asana and student, a variety of props can be used for the restorative practice. Bolsters, blankets, blocks, eye bags, yoga straps, chairs, sandbags and benches are some of the main types. If you plan to teach restorative yoga, you will need to either be in a studio that provides these props, have students provide their own props or have your own supply. The most basic are bolsters, blankets, yoga straps, blocks, and eye bags. (I prefer high-quality Mexican yoga blankets, but there are wool and others that work well also.) You will find your own preferences for props as you become more familiar with the practice. Bolsters come in a variety of shapes, sizes and firmness. Remember to plan for different body types and abilities.

Sticky Mats

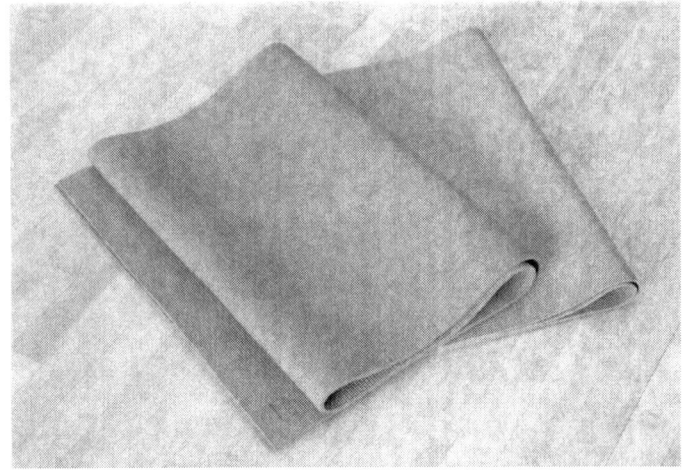

Blanket

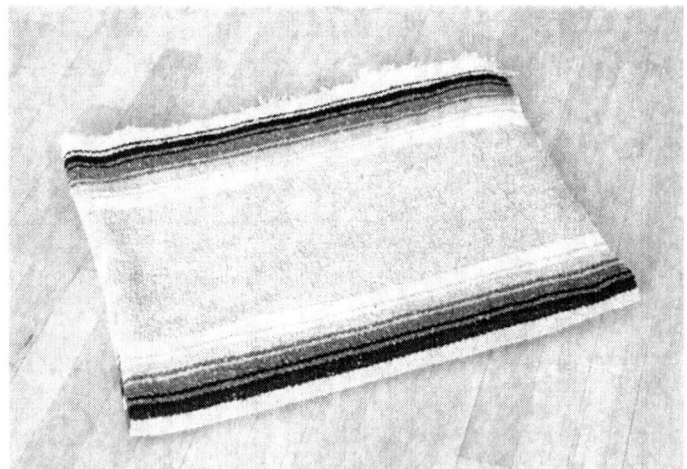

Small Cushions

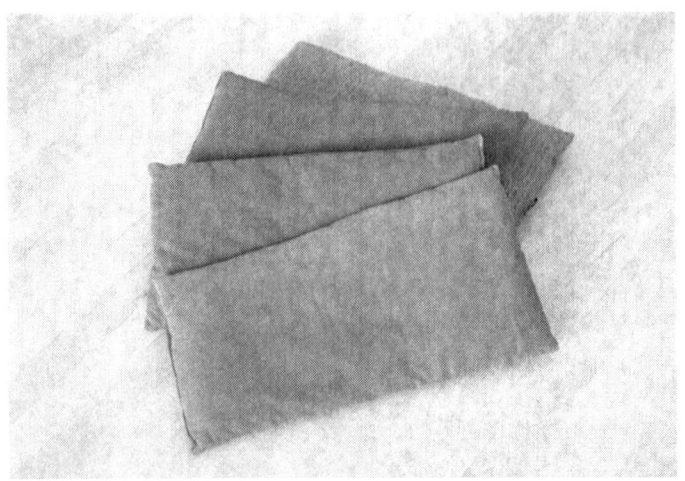

Bolsters

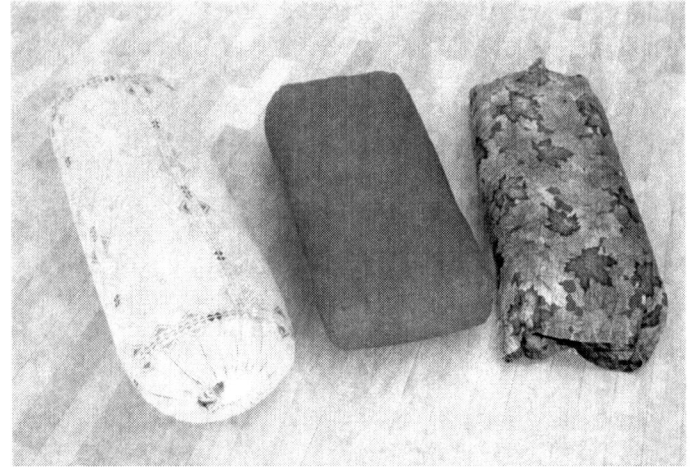

Small Table

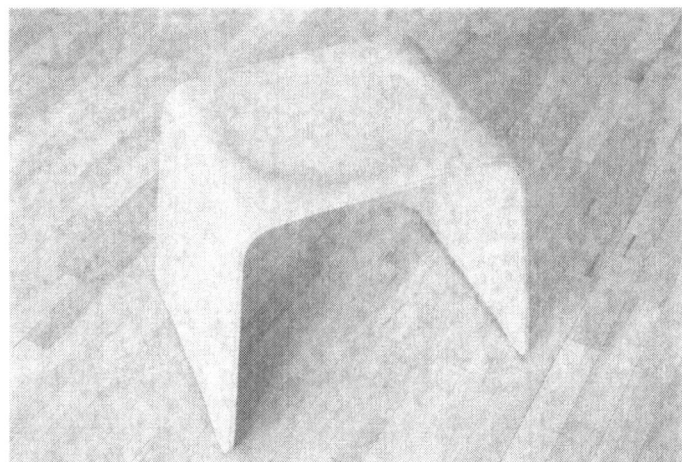

Yoga Chair

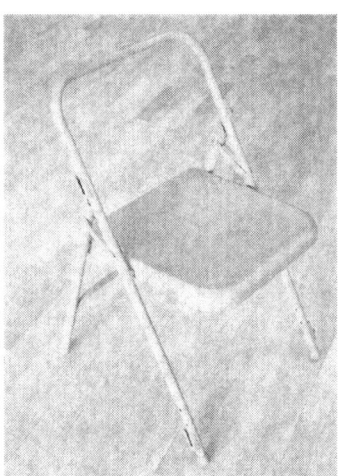

Straps

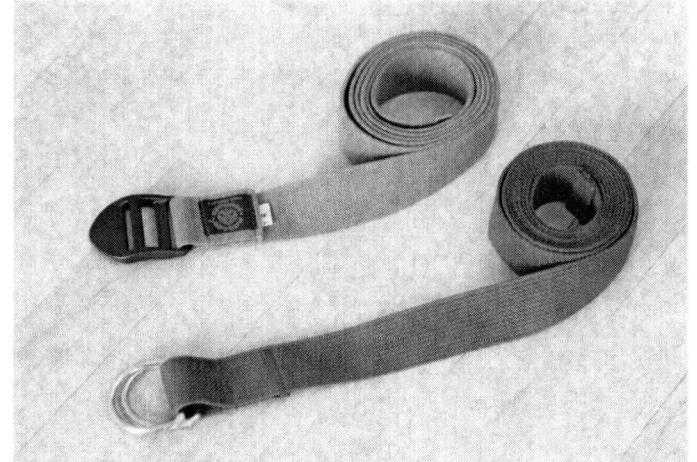

Eye Bags

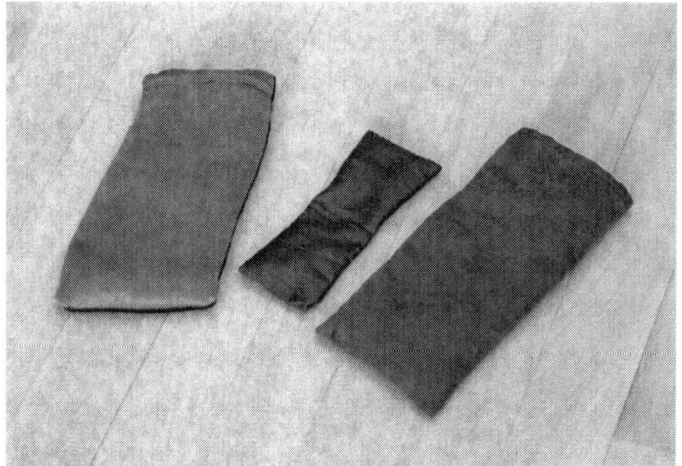

Blocks

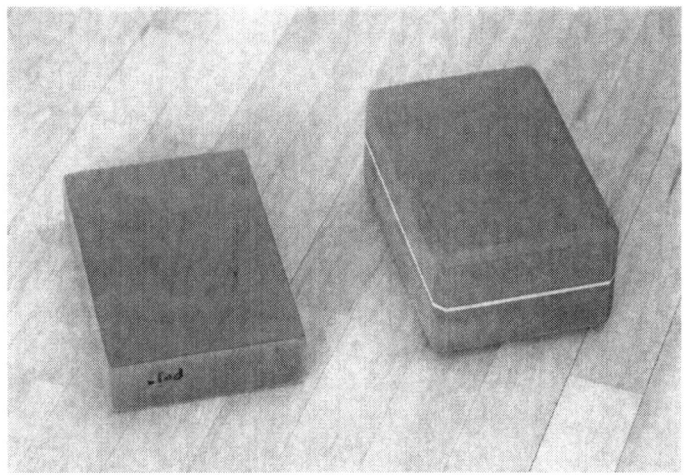

Organization of Students, Props and Space

The restorative practice often requires taking all the toys out of the closet, so to speak, and the studio can become quite full of props. If you know in advance what postures you will be practicing, instruct your students to gather the most likely props for that session. Each student will learn as they practice what extra props they may or may not need for their practice. I usually keep a variety of props at my side to use as needed when assisting my students. You may have already guessed: Restorative class can keep you very busy as a teacher–adjusting props, providing hands-on assists, reassuring the inexperienced and remaining attentive to the whole group.

Observation and Reading of Students

When you observe your students in their poses, you are gathering information to help serve them more fully. It is very important that your students are truly pain free when they are resting in their asanas. If they are trying to rest in a restorative posture, and are experiencing discomfort, they will not be able to rest. Their minds will keep coming back to the discomfort and grow agitated. If they are not comfortable, however, there is always a variation, or if necessary another pose. There can be situations where discomfort cannot be avoided. If the discomfort is not too great the student may relax around it and remain in the position, and the holding time may be decreased. This must be monitored and assessed individually.

Keen observation of your students is an important part of your teaching of restorative yoga. Are they relaxed or grimacing? Look carefully at the expressions on the faces of your students. If there is tension or wincing in some faces, invite the whole class to relax by saying, "relax your face," "soften your jaw," etc. Notice whether they shift. If not, check in with them personally and help them to make the appropriate adjustments. Sometimes the problem goes deeper than just tension in the jaw; the jaw may be just a mirror for greater discomfort that needs to be addressed. Observe their bodies. Do you note tension in one or more areas of their body or one side of their body in comparison to the other?

Allow your observation of your students to inform you about next steps. That can include what to say to the class as a whole. When your students are resting, that is a moment to teach them about the benefits of relaxation or about the specific posture and how it might apply to them, how to work with their minds or whatever other teaching that is appropriate in the moment. Be sure to also give them silence in which to rest as called for. Too much talk can be intrusive.

Also look for alignment of their props and bodies as they rest. Always prop both sides of the body, even if only one side is bothering them. This technique keeps the body in balance. (You can prop one side more fully than the other if need be.) Make sure they are resting evenly on top of their bolsters. Look at their feet, pelvis, shoulders, neck and head and check for alignment. Be alert and open to all the messages coming to you through your senses and your intuition.

Energetics of Alignment

Alignment can affect the flow of energy in each position. Yoga asanas can be seen as sacred geometry. An equilateral triangle has a different energy flow than a square, for example, or a straight line or curved one. If you were to run as fast as you can in a straight line you would find that you would use different muscles and thought patterns to go from point A to point B. While running on a curve you would have to adjust, putting more attention on one set of muscles. Energy flows, it just flows differently in different position and can be blocked or opened by different movements, angles, positions or asanas.

We also have the polarities of negative and positive, feminine and masculine and the chakras and nadis that can all be affected by our practice and alignment in our supported positions. When we connect our feet or our hands we are creating a connection of sun and moon, feminine and masculine, yin and yang, and a balancing of those energies in our being. When the feet are uneven or the hands not aligned this can be felt not only physically but energetically.

CHAPTER 5

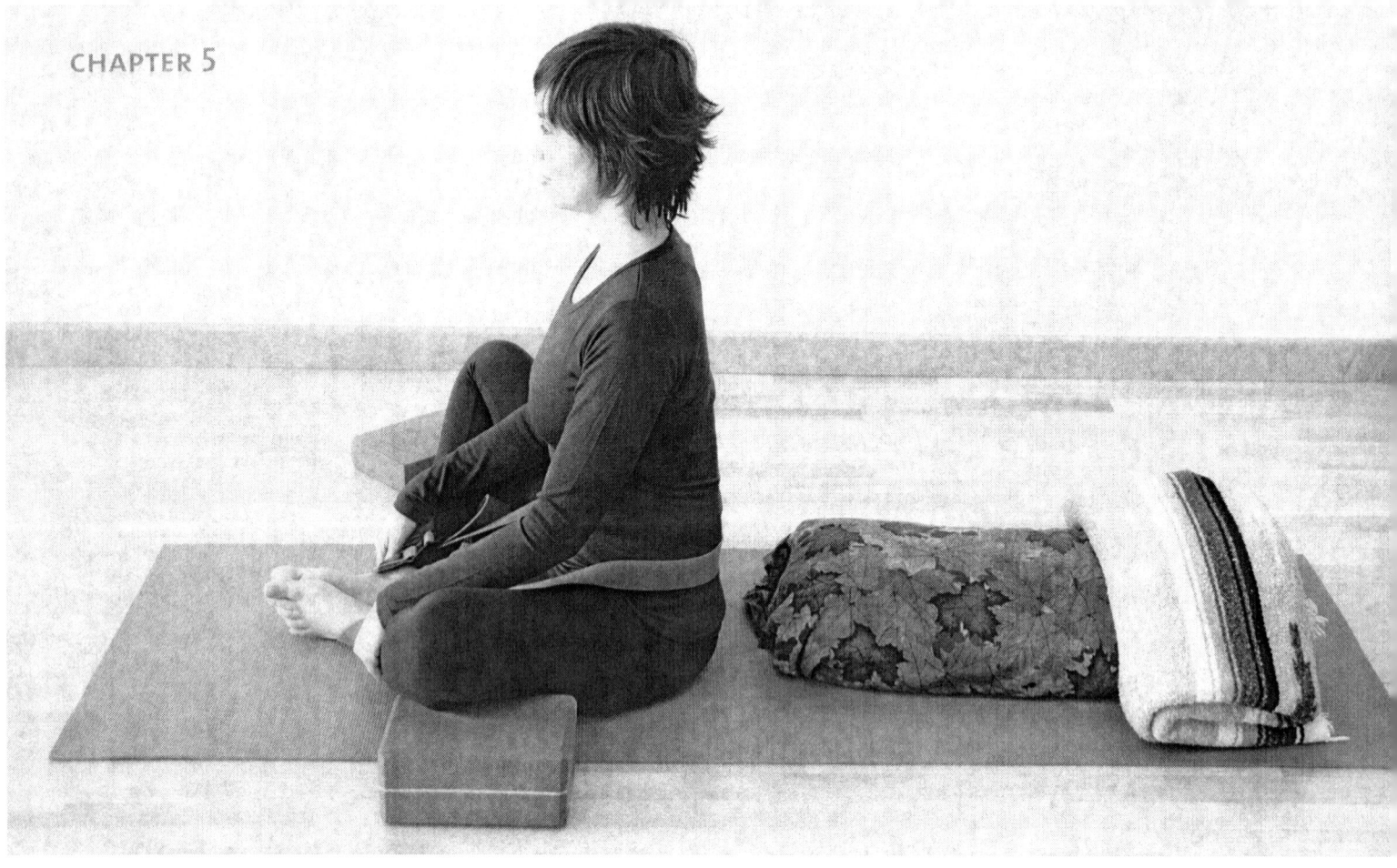

Warm-ups to Prepare for Your Restorative Flow

"For fast-acting relief, try slowing down."
Lily Tomlin

Creating Your Warm-up Flow

You can prepare your students for entering their restorative practice with a simple warm-up sequence or move directly into your restorative sequence. If they are more advanced students, the warm-ups can be more demanding including sun salutations, standing asanas, inversions, etc. Depending on the level of your class sometimes a more vigorous sequence can pave the way for the ability to relax more fully. If you are working with students who experience more limited mobility, tailor the warm-up to their conditions. Warm-ups should also be related to what you plan to teach during the resting section of your class and to address your students' particular needs. In classes of from 1 and 1/4 to 2 hours, I take from 15 to 30 minutes for meditation and warm-ups, and the remaining minutes are dedicated to a restorative flow. This can be adjusted according to the abilities and requirements of your students.

You can also use restorative poses to begin a session of asanas as a way to rest before entering a more active practice. Personally, at times if I am feeling very tired I will begin with one, two or three restorative postures and then move on to a more vigorous practice. Then I will finish with savasana. Another option is at the end of a normal asana sequence you can insert one or more restoratives before savasana.

Here is a general "Warm-Up Series" that I sometimes use right after the seated opening meditation that addresses gently opening the body from the head to feet. Your students may begin seated in a simple cross-legged position with support under the pelvis if needed in the center of room, or they can also be seated against the wall if back support is required. Use this series or create your own. Keep in mind the level of the class, the ability of the students and what restorative sequence you will be using.

Simple Neck Stretches: Allow the head to drop forward and relax around any areas holding tension for one to three complete breaths, then return to center. Allow the head to drop back, opening the throat, on an exhalation; on the inhale, lift the head to center. (If your student is sitting next to the wall have them move their head towards the wall. If they can touch the wall with their head they may relax their heads against the wall; if they are unable to reach the wall they can go as far as they can comfortably.) Gently drop the head to the right for one to three breaths and then repeat on the left side.

Simple Shoulder Rolls: Roll the shoulders up, back and around, coordinating the movement with breath. Inhale and take the shoulders up toward the ears; exhale, take the shoulders down and back around. In the opposite direction, inhale, take the shoulders back and up; exhale, release them forward and down.

Torso Circles: Seated in a cross-legged position, with hands resting on the knees and keeping the torso upright, moving from the hips circle the torso first in one direction and then in the other.

Upavista Konasana, Baddha Konasana, Dandasana Combo: I learned this sequence from Rodney Yee. Open the legs into Upavista Konasana (Seated Wide Angle Pose) and extending the legs, press down through the knees and out through the heels, keeping the legs active. Flex and point the feet together and alternately. Place the hands in prayer position and moving the feet together, bring the feet into Baddha Konasana (Cobbler's Pose), and then with the hands remaining in prayer position extend the feet out in front to Dandasana (Staff Pose). Place the fingertips slightly behind the pelvis, lift the sternum, place your shoulder blades onto your back by drawing your shoulder blades gently closer to each other, and elongate the spine. Depending on your students and time each of these asanas can be explored further as part of your warm-up series. For students with limited mobility, flexibility or strength the hands can remain on the floor to support the transitions between the postures.

Cat Cow on all fours in Table position: With the hands and knees on the floor, knees hip-width apart, flex the spine up, inhaling, and down, exhaling. Continue to coordinate the movement with the breath. Then open the spine laterally from side to side keeping the thighs perpendicular to the floor and moving the shoulder and pelvis towards each other from side to side and moving the head around to look at the hip on each side. Inhale when moving through center, exhale as you turn your head and hips toward each other. Come back to center. The hips may also be circled in both directions pausing for one or two breaths where there is holding and softening around any sensations.

Adho Mukha Svanasana (Downward-Facing Dog): From table position take the buttocks back to the heels and extend the arms overhead on the floor; plant the hands on the floor without pulling them under your shoulders and come back into your table position, and extend the legs while raising the coccyx up towards the sky. Pull the thighs back toward the wall behind you, breathe, alternate one heel moving towards the floor and the other leg bending at the knee. For more flexible students draw the heels towards the floor and lift the toes.

Add or delete any posture that will support your students more fully. Now you are ready to move into your restorative sequence.

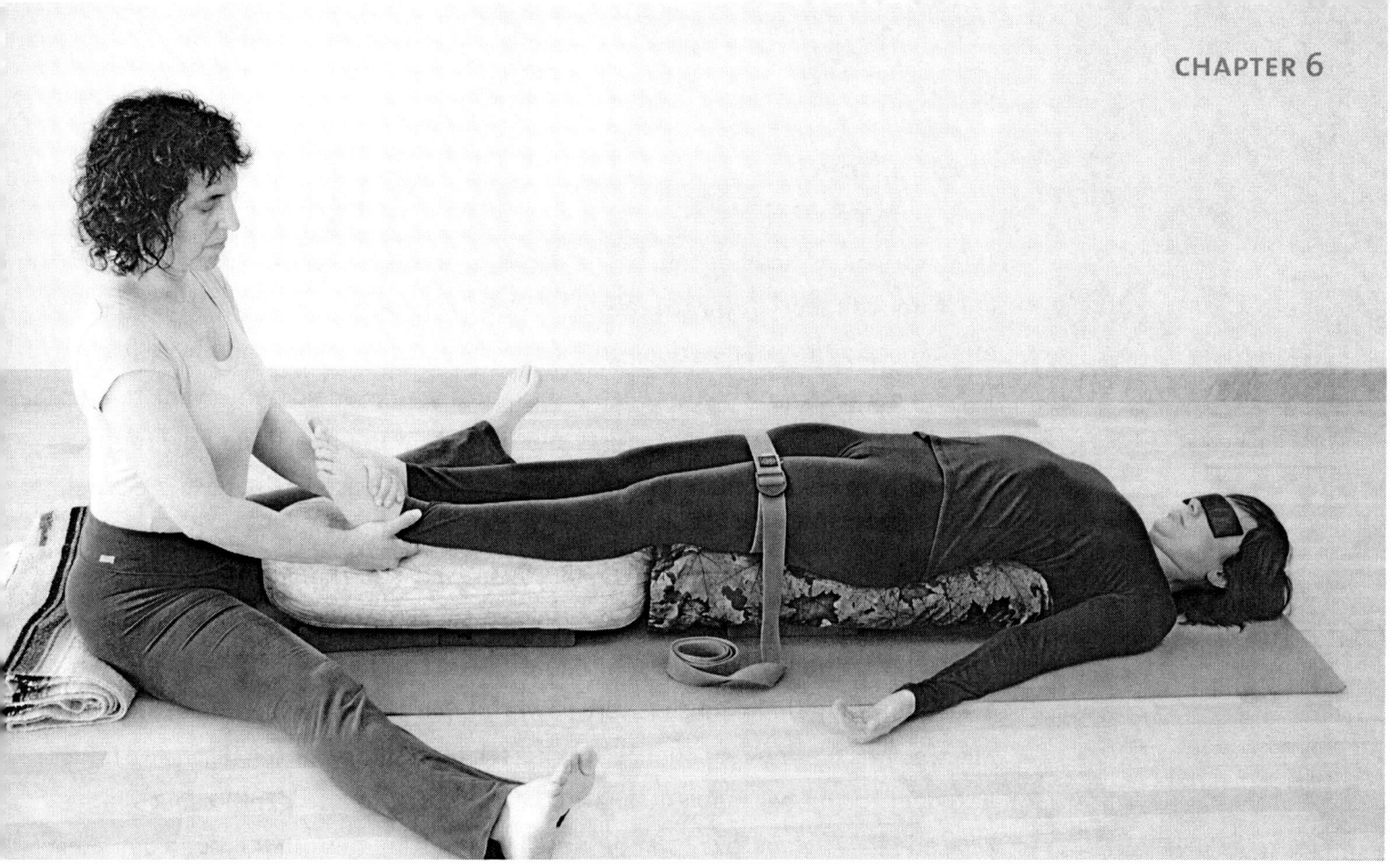

Postures and Hands-on Adjustments

Touching Students with Consciousness

Every body is sacred. This is the attitude I take when touching my students. I think, "This being is precious," and so when I touch them physically or energetically, I touch them with the utmost respect and care. Let your students know you will be touching them and make sure that it is okay with them if you have any doubt. The first time you work with someone ask their permission. "I will be doing some hands-on assists, is that okay with you?" or something similar. If they say no, respect that fully. As they gain your trust you can ask them again. I have had very few students who have requested I don't touch them, but if they do not want to be touched I honor that fully.

"Too often we underestimate the power of a touch, a smile, a kind word, a listening ear, an honest compliment, or the smallest act of caring, all of which have the potential to turn a life around." Leo Buscaglia

Kinds of Touch

There are many kinds of touch. The depth of touch is one important aspect of touch. You can touch firmly, deeply, lightly, with confidence, timidly. All this is being communicated to your student on a tissue level, feeling level and physical level. The energy with which you touch also affects your students. You want to help them to relax when you give assists and help them to understand how to move their body to create greater alignment, opening and ease in the position. When you touch them watch for their reaction. Become ultra sensitive to them so you can perceive what is going on and adjust your assist accordingly. What is the reason you are touching your students? Where are you coming from? As a teacher we have a responsibility to understand how we are touching our students and why are we touching them. Touch is very powerful. Our present perceptions can be influenced by a previous experience. Touch is felt in the moment, but it can also bring a student to another moment. I have given an assist to a student in a restorative pose and they began to cry. Not because I was hurting them, but I found out later that they became in touch with the loss of a loved one when I touched them. We must realize that while touch can be felt in this moment it can also bring a student into a past memory or experience, and into deep peace and relaxation as well.

Matching Touch with Students' Needs

Developing sensitivity to your students has several levels. One of my teachers, Amrit Desai, said, "The body is the most sacred temple you will ever come to." Keep this in mind when you are touching your students.

- What do you know about your students' conditions, and how can that inform you about their needs?
- Are they male or female? We need to respect the cultural norms for appropriate and inappropriate places to touch on both the female and male body.
- Do they have any injuries or postural tendencies?
- What is your intuition?
- What do you do if you are unsure? If you are unsure, take a breath, wait and don't touch until you have an understanding of why and how you are touching your student.

- What do you want to transmit with your touch? When you touch your student, open yourself with prayer or thoughts of healing, peace or the energy you want to transmit with your touch.

The Energetics of Touch

Everything is energy and has a vibration. When you touch your students you become a conduit of energy. What kind of energy do you want to transmit to your student? Is it healing, loving or compassionate energy? Become conscious of the energy you are transmitting when touching your student. Are you thinking about what you are going to do after class as you are pulling on their neck? Connect your touch with your thoughts and then allow the energy to flow through you to your student. Become a channel allowing only goodness to move through you. Bring yourself as fully present as possible.

How to Protect Your Body and Energy When Assisting Students

When you are moving around your class and you sense a student with an unclear energy you may choose not to touch them. You may visualize energy moving from you to them but not allowing their energy to move toward you. You may surround yourself in white light while assisting them. You may visualize a barrier at your elbows that allows energy to move down your arms but not up; when their energy reaches your elbows it gets dispersed. You may also choose not to assist a particular student because you feel you will be adversely affected by touching them. This must also be honored.

When you are assisting, protect yourself by using correct body mechanics. Keep your back straight, and avoid leaning over your students to do an assist when you can be sitting or squatting next to them, bringing your center of gravity lower and keeping your back upright. Use your body weight to help you when appropriate.

The following are some techniques that you can use to clear your energy or the space where you have been giving your session or class. Use what resonates with you. Create your own ritual or do what feels good to you--these are just ideas. After teaching and touching your students, wash your hands or use another one of the following clearing techniques to clear your own energy. You can clear your personal energy and the energy of the room you are working in by using a mantra. Say or sing a mantra and allow its vibration to fill you and the room. This can be a sanskrit manta or you can repeat a word or a simple set of words in English. You can use a bell of some kind or a Tibetan singing bowl. Use your mind's intention coupled with a mantra or sound--clapping of hands, for example--to shift the energy. You can burn sage or incense, surrounding yourself with the smoke to clear your energy. Your intention and conscious acknowledgment of what you are creating will help you to shift and clear your energy.

Basic Assists

I have given a number of assists in the posture section of the book, Chapters 10 and 11. Below is an overview of some of the principle assists. These assists can be applied to a variety of poses depending on the positions.

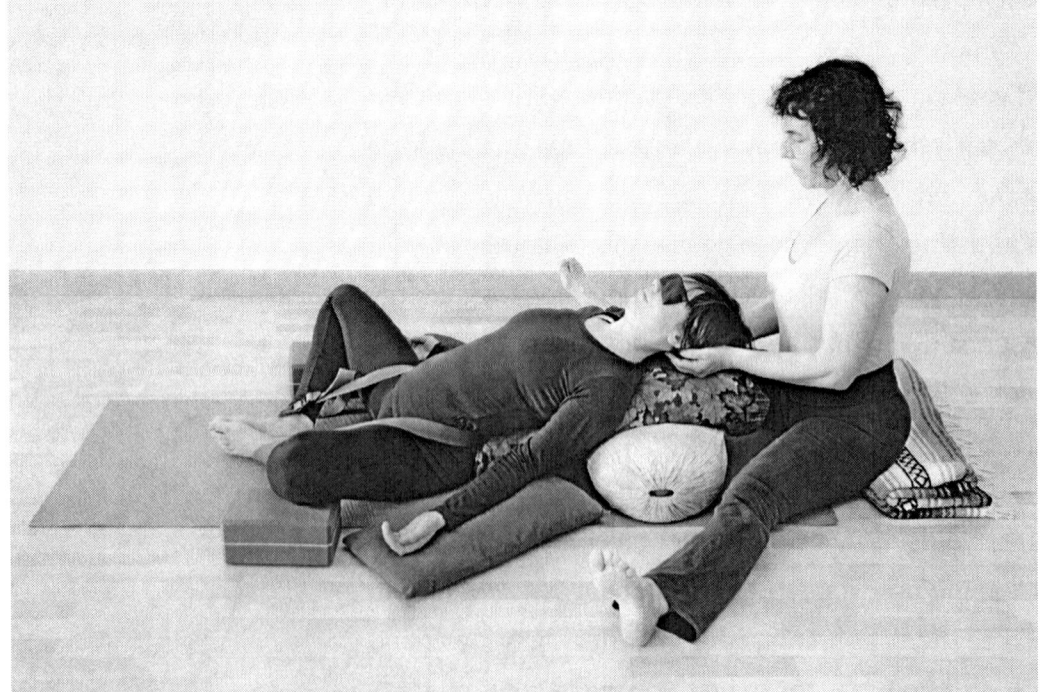

Head Hold: While students are resting simply take their head into your hands. Hold their head with almost no pressure and encourage them to relax their head into your hands. This can create profound relaxation. Be patient and feel their head little by little become heavier and release into your hands. Keep yourself and your hands relaxed.

Gentle Neck Pull: Take the student's head into your hands. Feel for where the skull meets the head. There is a ridge there on the bottom or edge of the skull. Place your fingertips gently under that ridge and pull the head towards you, elongating the back of the neck.

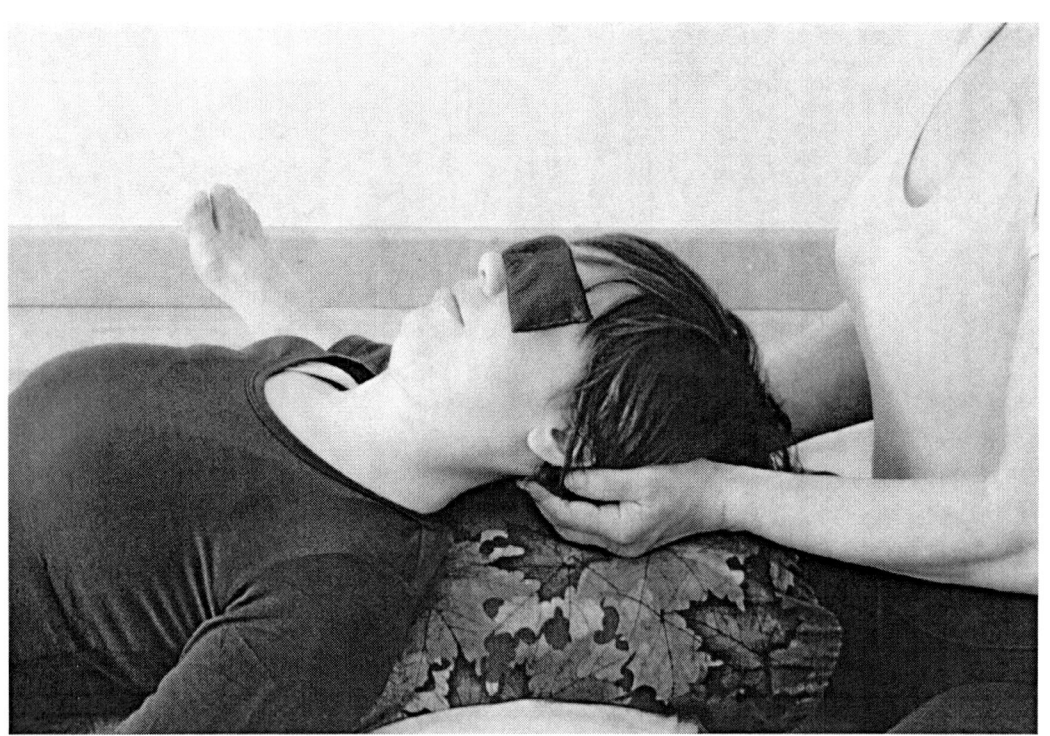

Three Points in Shoulder: There are three main pressure points where stress is habitually held in the tops of the shoulders that when pressed can release tensions, sometimes superficial, sometimes more profound. Sit with your pelvis supported if needed, at the student's head. If you are unsure where to press first feel the general area. Feel for where the bones are. The clavicle or collarbones are in the front. You are looking for three points in the fleshy part behind the collarbones towards the very top of the shoulder. Press your thumbs there starting close to the neck for the first point and then incrementally move out along the shoulder toward the arms for the second and third points. Feel the tissue and mus-

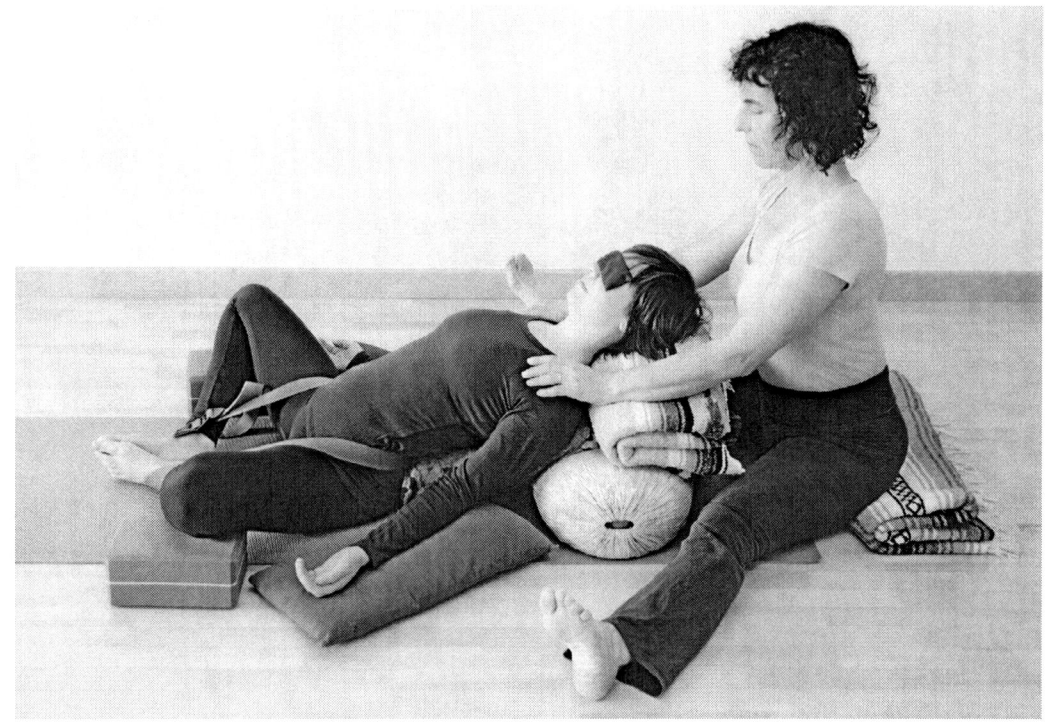

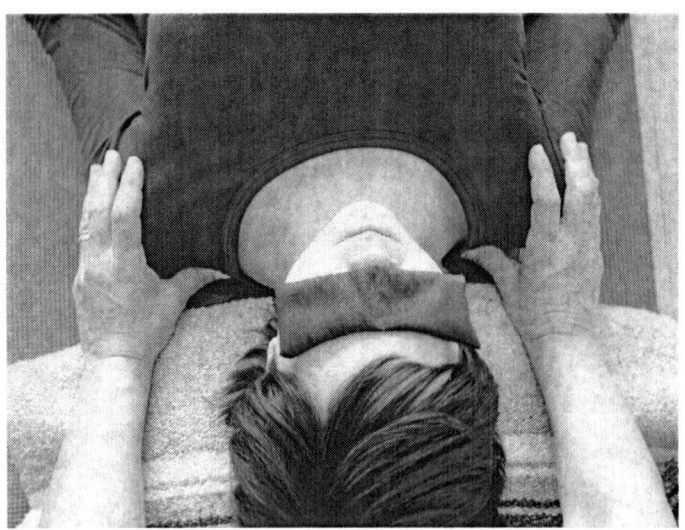 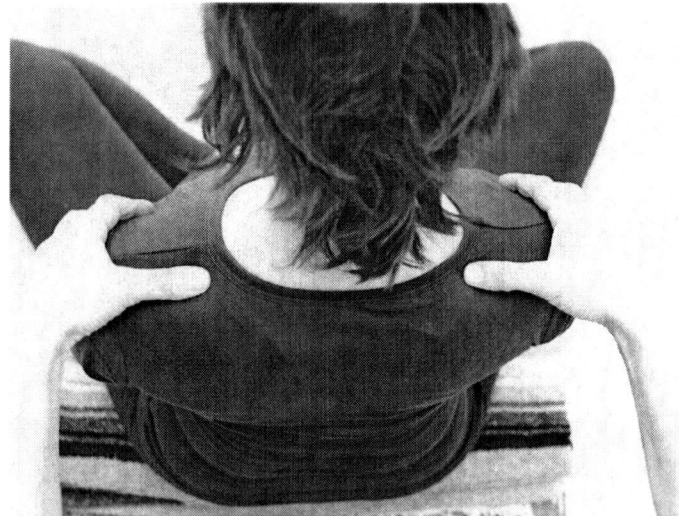

cle under your fingers. Notice if it is soft or hard. Begin by pressing gently until you feel the tissue soften, and you can then move in more deeply. You can spend up to four breaths on each point, increasing the pressure only if you feel the muscles soften.

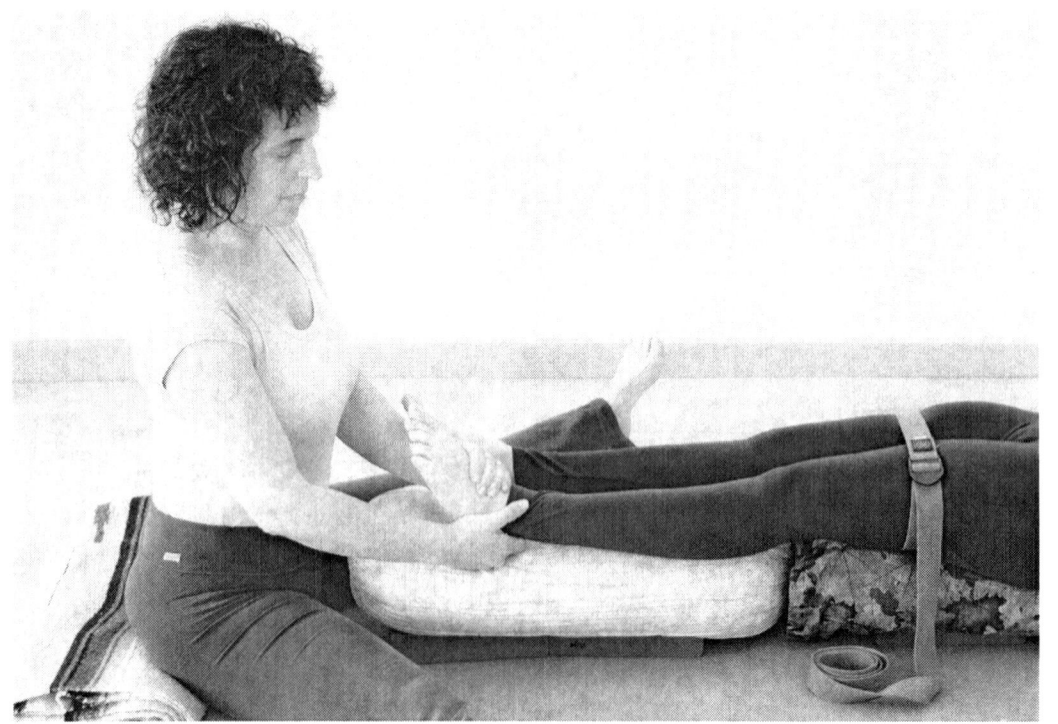

Foot Hold or Massage: This can be as simple as holding the foot or feet for a few moments. Take the sides of the foot into your hands for a moment or two or place one hand around the heel of the foot and the other on the top of the foot, hold and take one or several breaths depending on your time. Or for a more complex massage, make small circular motions with your thumb or knuckle over the sole of the foot— the arch, the center and the sides. Start from the ball of the foot near the toes and work your way down to the heel or start from the heel and move to the toes

Hand Hold or Massage: This can be as simple as holding the student's hand in your two hands and gently breathing. You can take it further, time permitting, by pressing on the palm of the hand with your thumbs, palm face up or with your finger tips, palms face down. You might massage each finger as well.

Massaging on Either Side of the Spine: From either a standing, seated or another position depending on the posture the student is in, place the thumbs or the heel of the hand on either side of the spine. Never press directly on the spine. Press into the muscles on either side of the spine. Move either from the shoulders to the low back or from the low back to shoulders.

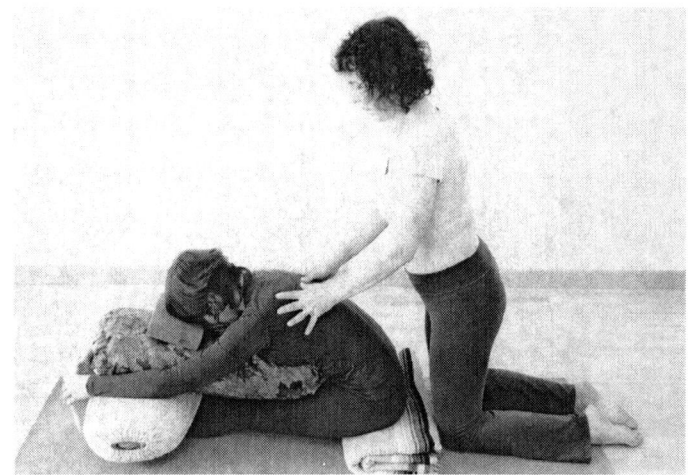

Low Back Press at an Angle: From behind the student, place the hands on either side of the low back with fingers facing down towards the floor (see photo right). While maintaining some pressure into the back, gently move the hands down in the direction of the floor on either side of the spine, to help it lengthen. The focus here is not to press the student farther forward but to elongate their spine and encourage a deeper surrender into the pose.

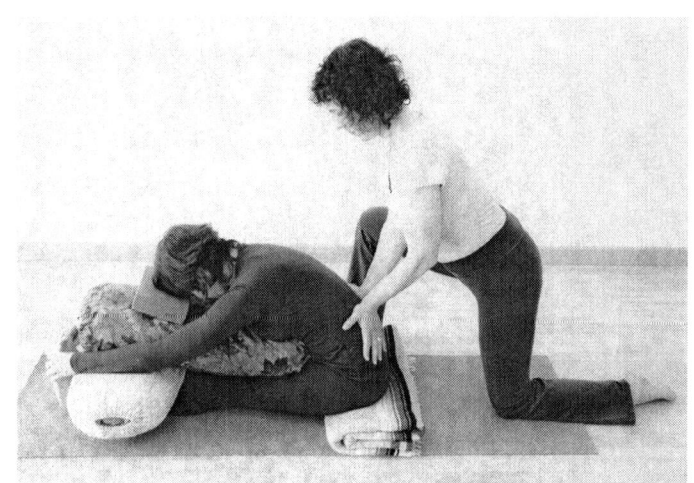

Back Press Downward: When your student is face down with their back parallel to the floor you may press the palms of your hands, making contact with the complete hand including fingers, on either side of their spine. Start at either end, from the shoulders and moving to the low back or starting at the low back and moving toward the shoulders.

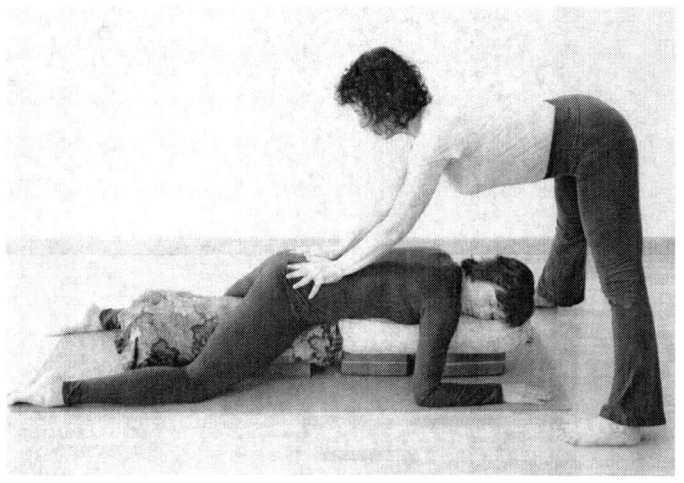

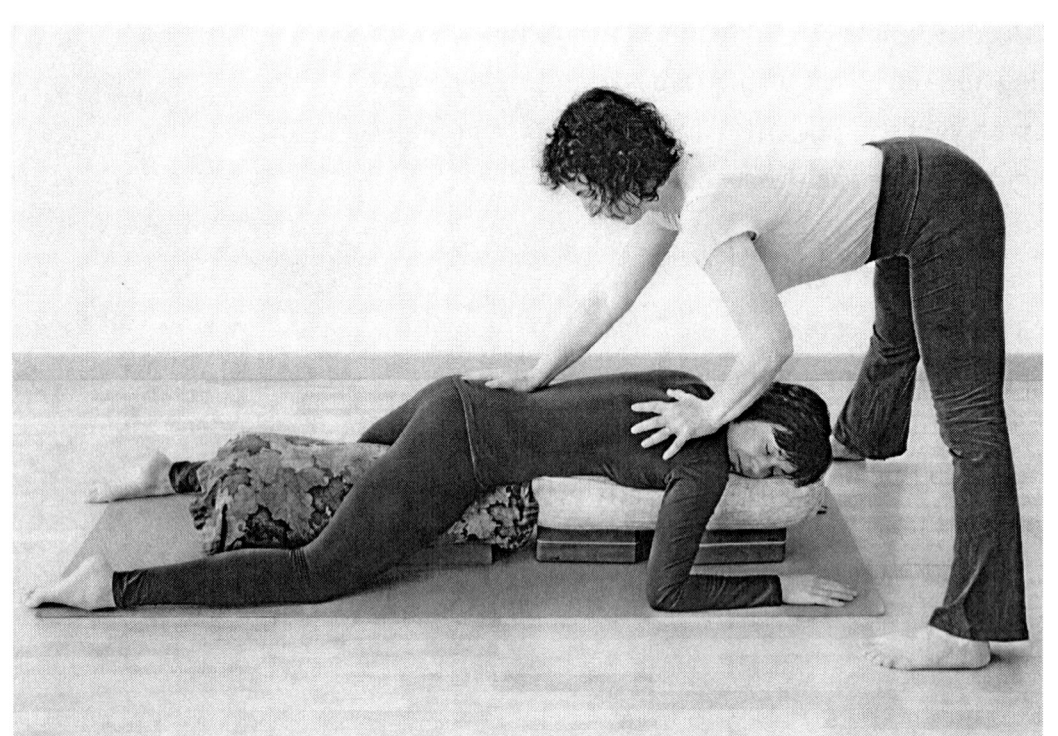

Diagonal Low Back Press: Place one hand on your student's shoulder and the other on the opposite side of the lower back. Press the hands gently down and away from each other at the same time. Repeat with the opposite side.

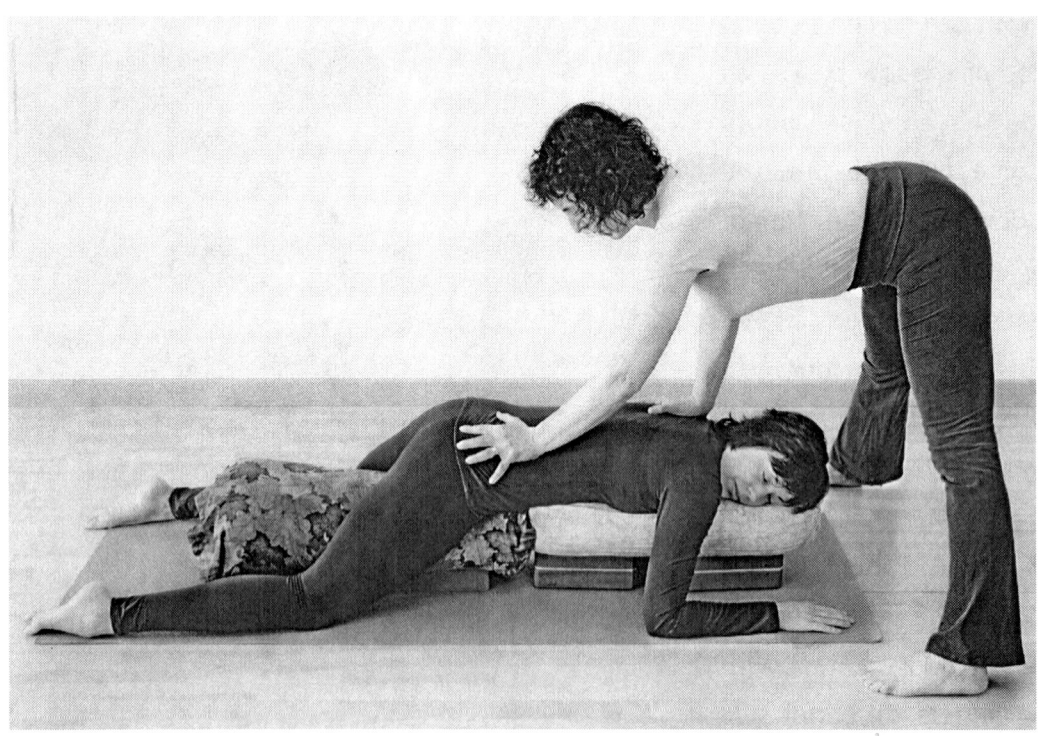

Heart to Neck Polarity: Lay one hand on the heart and one hand under the neck. Energy flows out the right and into the left so see and feel the movement of energy moving from the hands through the student's body up through your body and back around to theirs. Or simply breathe and allow the prana or energy to move where it needs to go.

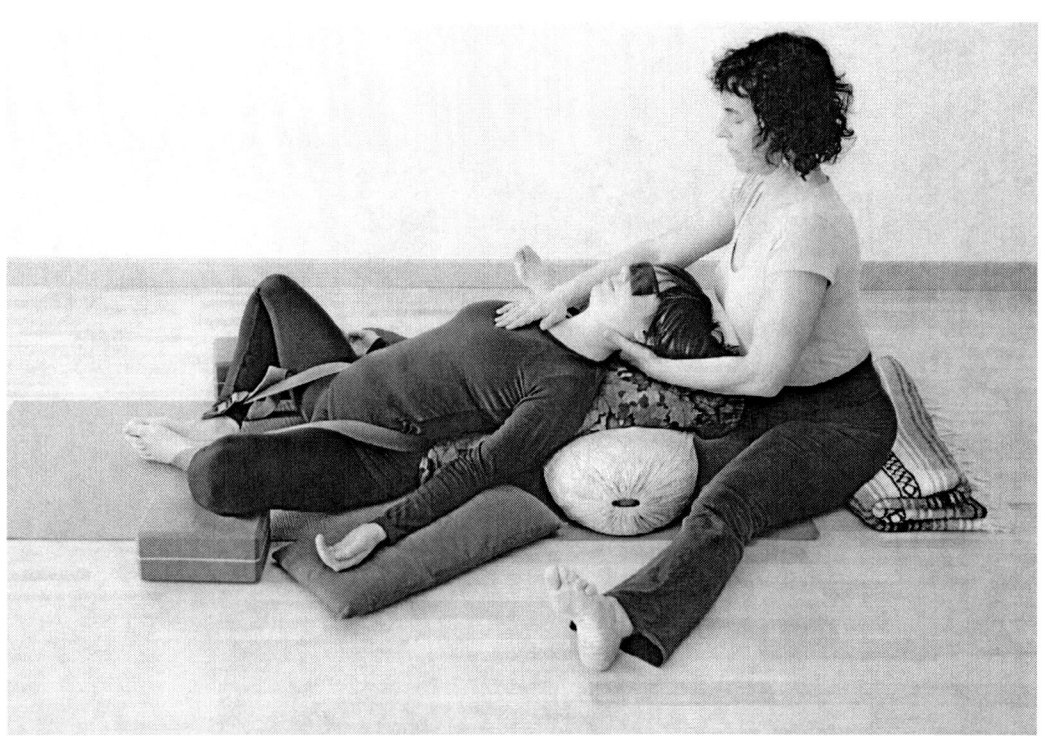

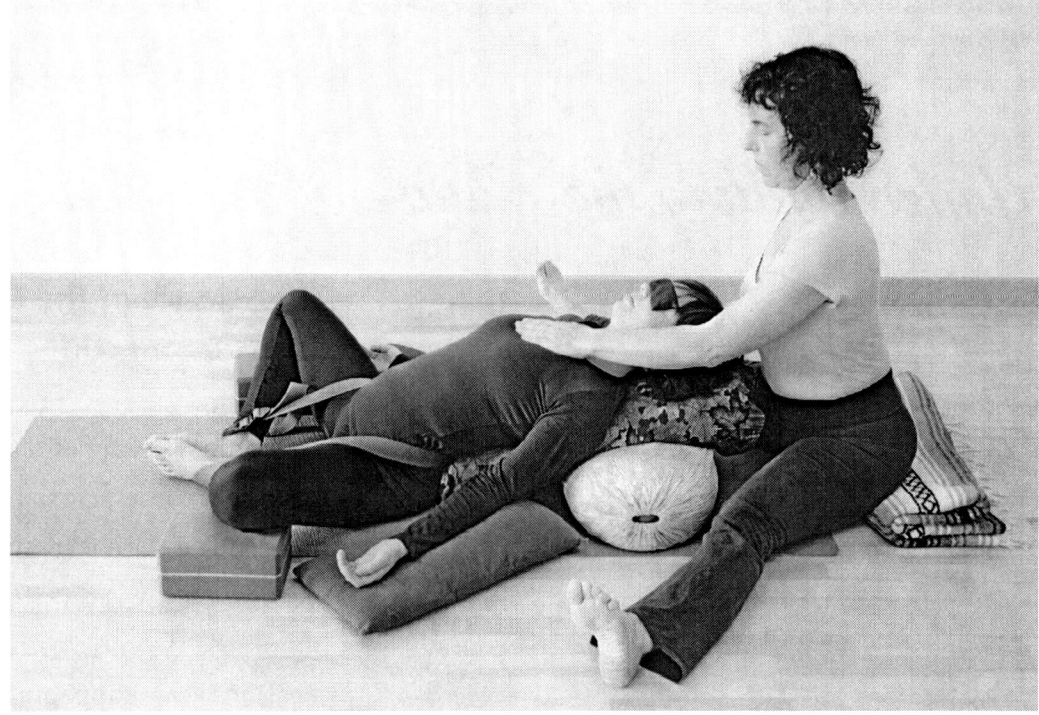

CHAPTER 7

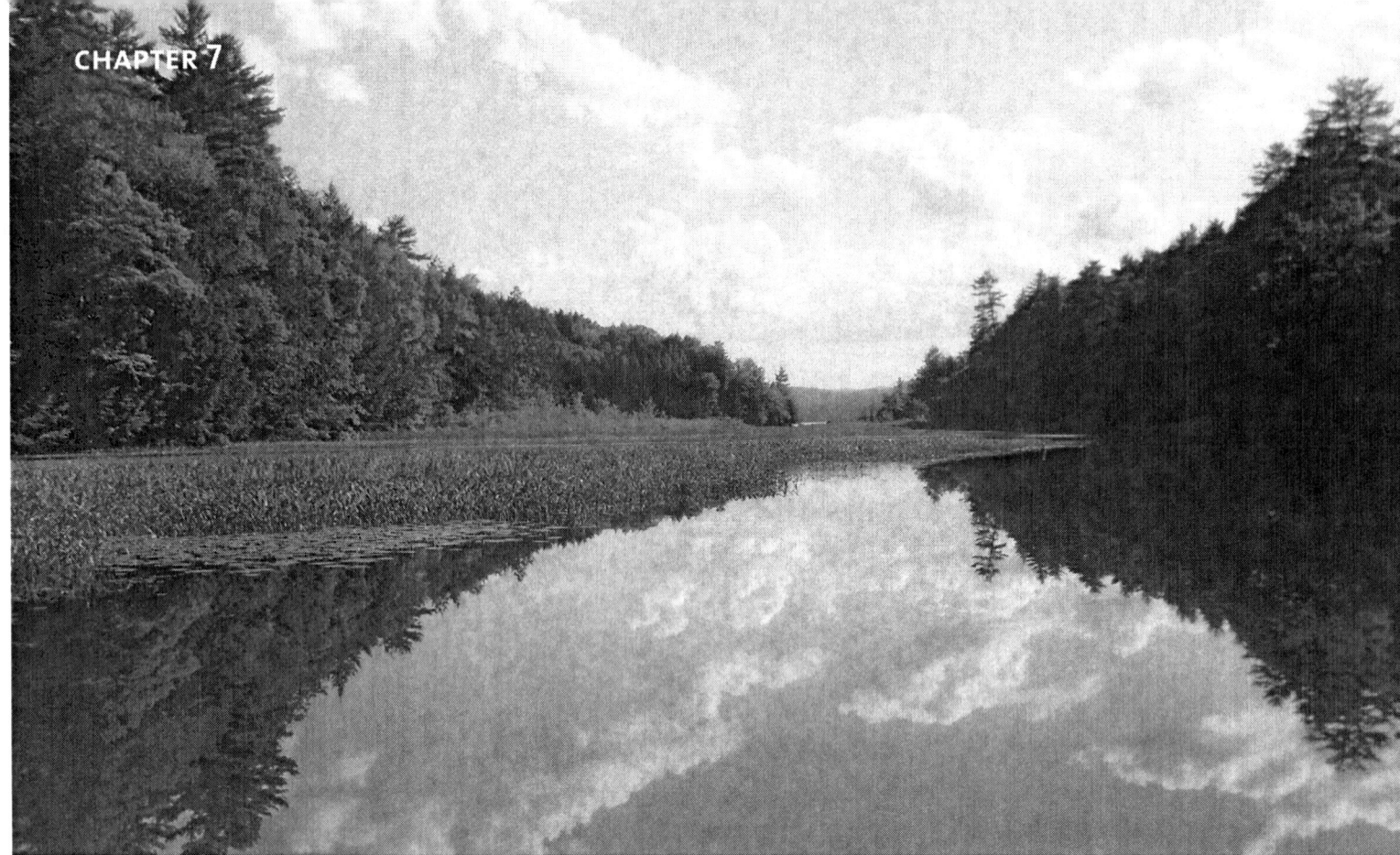

Photo by Sue Flamm

Understanding the Nature of the Mind

"Yoga is the cessation of the turnings of the mind."
The second aphorism of Patanjali's Yoga Sutras

The Science of the Body, Mind and Stress Connection

Each time we enter into a restorative resting pose, we inevitably come across the mind. When the mind is preoccupied with stressful thoughts, pain, or worldly worries, energy is diverted into these areas. Depending on the degree of stress, hormones and chemical reactions are happening that are being triggered from the mind. In more yogic terms vital energy gets caught up in these places and is not free to move; it can't revitalize other areas of our being that need attention. This is why it is important to understand how to work with the mind as an integral part of the practice.

There is now substantial research linking the mind and the immune system. It is now widely accepted that stress contributes to illness and that relaxation promotes a stronger immune system. Restorative Yoga is a system that teaches relaxation and support not only for the body but also for the mind. Stress is a big contributing factor to disease/dis-ease and distress in our fast-paced lives. The mind and body are intimately connected.

Mind defined by Deepack Chopra: *"The mind is an embodied and relational process that regulates the flow of energy and information. There is no mental event that does not have a neural correlate. There is no neural correlate that doesn't have a biological correlate. Everything in the body and mind is integrated."*

Let's look at how the brain or mind and the immune system interact. What makes sense to me intrinsically and intuitively has now become proven by science.

Stress can:
- Lower your immune system
- Increase heart disease risk factors such as hypertension and high cholesterol levels
- Cause you to eat in unhealthy ways in response to the stress
- Lead to depression
- Put you at a greater risk for heart disease, obesity and kidney dysfunction
- Trigger autoimmune diseases

Esther Sternberg has done extensive research on the physiological effects of stress on the body. When she refers to stress she talks about the physiological responses created in the body by external stress stimulus which include a feeling of increased anxiety, increased heart rate, tightening of muscles, sweating and having the urge to urinate. These responses can be triggered by countless events. Along with these external events or symptoms, inside the body hormones and chemical interactions are also happening. The human body is programmed to fight or run as a means of survival. This well-known fight-or-flight response when we are presented with danger can save our lives in certain situations, but the problem now is that we are increasingly triggering this reaction. We have to understand that it is not just the situation at hand but also our perception of the danger or perception of the situation that also affects the stress response. We cannot control most of the life events and situations that come our way each day. That is life and we on some level accept that. Sometimes all flows well and at other times stressful situations arise. If there is a stress-filled event that happens and we have time to recover then there is no real effect on our immune system. Even if there are several events with time to recover in between our bodies can handle that. It is when we have a constant stressful situation like caring for someone with Alzheimer's or another chronic disease, or a series of stressful events one after the other or perceived continual stressful events that we can run into trouble. The unfortunate truth is that many of us are dealing with chronic stress that is becoming more the norm than the exception.

What is the connection between the mind/brain and the immune response? When we are constantly stressed we begin to rapid-fire certain stress hormones, and certain nerve chemicals get activated that decrease the immune system's ability to fight disease. The brain's stress center, the hypothalamus, pumps out a hormone that causes the adrenal gland to pump out cortisol (which you may have heard of as cortisone cream--an anti-inflammatory cream used for poison ivy and other topical swelling), which is one of the most potent anti-inflammatory drugs that the body makes. What you may not be aware of is that this hormone is supposed to be released with stress, but then cease after the stressful situation is over. What happens with prolonged or chronic stress is that it is being secreted more often and sometimes consistently. While cortisol is being secreted the immune system and function is being inhibited. This can lead to more serious health problems. Some of the health problems are anti-inflammatory and autoimmune diseases including chronic fatigue syndrome, lupus, rheumatoid arthritis and many others. Being stressed consistently can also lead to being tired and to depression. Being stressed does not cause cancer but can block the body's ability to fight off certain cancers and other more simple illnesses like the common cold or flu.

The restorative practice as explained in this book helps to counteract these potentially debilitating effects on the body, mind and emotions. It has now been proven that yoga, tai chi, prayer, meditation, gentle exercise and the placebo effect can create a mental state that counteracts the state that stress creates. These practices release counteracting hormonal and chemical reactions in the brain and body that bring healing and peace to the practitioner.

When we rest in a restorative posture and experience physical discomfort, we are usually not able to rest for long, because our minds keep coming back to the discomfort. Instead of resting, the mind becomes even more agitated. For this reason, any discomfort in a pose should be immediately addressed with adjustments or variations. After the physical concerns are addressed, the mind must also be addressed.

If a student has constant pain because of a physical condition, he or she can learn to work with this pain through their asana practice, using support and variations. Having chronic pain is stressful in itself. Through the restorative practice they can learn about how to relax around the pain and also how to accept the pain. We use the word "practice" frequently in the yoga world; this is because we practice with consciousness on the mat so that we can bring this learning and the realizations into our daily lives. It is equally important that the student learns to work with the mental components of the constant pain, along with the physical ones.

Understanding the Nature of the Mind From a Yogic Perspective

This issue is very simple and very complex at the same time. To begin with, trying to understand the mind with the mind goes beyond the scope of what the mind (as we usually understand it) can grasp. The mind is limited in its ability to think outside of its belief systems and constructs. After all, it has created those systems in an attempt to make sense of what it perceives as its world. These perceptions and beliefs aren't always accurate or reliable, but they are usually deeply entrenched and taken for granted.

Mind, as I'm using it here, is a vast and "self" protective repository of memory, story and emotion. It is heavily influenced by the past, including past interpretations of its experiences, and has little ability to think beyond its own filters. In that sense, it is quite limited. It can have trouble perceiving situations directly, because it's attached to its own stories and beliefs about what is true. Mind can only exist in the past or the future (breath and body exist in the moment).

Whereas a conditioned mind does not usually perceive life directly because of its habitual filters, there is a consciousness available to everyone that is free of conditioning. Sometimes called "witness consciousness," this open and unobstructed capacity can see and feel what is, rather than identifying with our emotions and patterns and believing them to be who we are in any moment.

Witness consciousness can see the activities of mind for what they are. When we are not in witness consciousness we can be identifying with our problems and pain and believing that we are that problem or pain. When we identify with our suffering as who we are in that moment we lose sight of the bigger picture and can believe that we are that suffering. We are not our minds nor are we our bodies. When we can disconnect in this way we are able to also disconnect from the stressful thoughts and feelings and short circuit the stress cycle.

Mindfulness

Mindfulness is a Buddhist practice that can be applied to the restorative practice. It is being present with all that is happening inside of you at any given moment and embracing it with acceptance and compassion. Bringing mindfulness, acceptance and compassion into our practice helps us to relax even more fully. When the mind begins to entertain the thoughts and judgments such as, "my mind should be quiet …I should be feeling peaceful…. I should be feeling more comfortable… I shouldn't be thinking about this or that," it all creates separation from the reality of what is. Creating space to receive all of who you are in any moment is an absolute gift. Encourage your students to create space to receive themselves and bring mindfulness into their restorative practice.

"Feelings, whether of compassion or irritation, should be welcomed, recognized, and treated on an absolutely equal basis; because both are ourselves. The tangerine I am eating is me. The mustard greens I am planting are me. I plant with all my heart and mind. I clean this teapot with the kind of attention I would have were I giving the baby Buddha or Jesus a bath. Nothing should be treated more carefully than anything else. In mindfulness, compassion, irritation, mustard green plant, and teapot are all sacred." The Miracle of Mindfulness: An Introduction to the Practice of Meditation, Thich Nhat Hanh

Looking at the Mind from a Quantum Perspective

As I've said before, we live in a vibrational world. Every being – plant, insect, animal, mineral – carries a vibration. Every cell and molecule has a vibration. The mind is powerful, because every thought that we think also carries a vibration. Dr Masaru Emoto, author of *The Hidden Messages in Water*, has performed some amazing studies on the effect of directing thoughts, words, music or emotions into water. He found when taking photos of the water in frozen crystalline form, that the water with positive, loving thoughts directed towards it made beautiful, unique, symmetrical snowflake-like patterns in the water. When negative thoughts were directed into the water, there were asymmetrical or chaotic patterns in the frozen crystals.

This information is relevant to our discussion, because it shows how powerful our thoughts are. If you take a moment to reflect on the fact that more than half of the human body is made up of water, you begin to catch a glimpse of the important connection between mind and body. Just imagine the effect your thoughts might have on the water that you are made up of. Think of the power you have over supporting the functioning of the fluid in your body. Our thoughts have the potential to affect our internal makeup. Remembering that we are not our thoughts, but the vibration of our thoughts affects our body and being. Thoughts create neuron reactions in the brain. When we practice thinking over and over certain kinds of thought patterns, for example, "I am not enough," like working a muscle we strengthen these patterns and neural pathways and these thought pathways become neural highways; so in order to break into new pathways of thinking we have to do the work of cutting down the trees, making a new path and eventually paving the road to a new superhighway that takes us into a healthful relationship with ourselves and our world around us.

Now of course there are other things to consider, such as individual constitution and environmental factors, for example, but we as individuals can, nevertheless, affect our health through the choices we make. Operating from a calm, open mind helps us see our choices more clearly. One of those choices is the mental diet we create. That is, we can affect our inner state on several levels with our attachment to positive or negative thoughts.

Mind-Emotion Connection

Take a moment to reflect - what do you think comes first, thought or emotion? One of the teachers who has helped me to work with my mind is Byron Katie. In her book, *Loving What Is*, she explains how our thoughts create our emotional reactions, and our reactions further reinforce what we think. Without examining the mental diet we feed on, we can't fully understand our own experiences, and we have little in the way of creating true, clear choices. As we become more present to "what is," we can begin to let go of stressful, even debilitating, thinking and emotional patterns.

Staying Out of Your Personal Story

Help your students to understand this. We all have our personal story, trauma, successes and failures. We all have ingrained patterns and habits. When you can notice that you are entering your story take a step back. All we truly have is this moment, nothing more, nothing less. Is it serving you to continue following your story? Dropping into the moment we face what is there for us now. Just as what we meet with on the yoga mat and in our practice is a metaphor for our lives, our thought patterns and habits also appear on the mat, at work, driving in the car and lying in bed at night. The difference is that when we are on the mat we have the opportunity to be conscious of our patterns and habits. Acknowledge your story - you might cry - but be willing to entertain the possibility of dropping your story. Who would you be without your story and all that you feel and think around it? Stories can become habitual ways of thinking and feeling and can repeat over and over. When we observe our minds we come to discover the reccurring patterns that can be guiding forces for our lives. When we become conscious of this we can begin to liberate ourselves from the hold of our limiting beliefs. The following are some techniques to work with the mind. Each of them can reduce stress and increase a place for calm and peace.

These methods have helped hundreds of my students to release stress. It has now been scientifically proven that they reduce cortisol levels and help to balance the effects of stress. Many lifestyle-changing programs include one or more of these techniques to help people live a healthier life.

Linking Breath with Thoughts

I like to use this technique when my students are resting in their poses or in seated meditation. "Breathe in loving kindness and compassion, breathe out loving kindness and compassion," or "Breathe in relaxation and healing, breathe out dis-ease and distress." Another teacher of mine, Thich Nhat Hanh, in his book *The Blooming of a Lotus*, suggests many meditations using the idea of linking thought and breath.

Always with a compassionate attitude:
Breathe in what we want to cultivate and breathe out what we want to release.
Breathing in and out what we want to cultivate.
Breathe in and out simply becoming present with our reality of what is without judgment.
Breathe in and out with compassion the uncomfortable things that we experience or that others experience to cultivate compassion for all those on the planet or for someone we know who is struggling with this in his or her life. This is a powerful form of Tonglen, a Buddhist meditation practice.

Meditation is certainly a large topic, but we can intervene on our own behalf more simply than we sometimes imagine. A few slow breaths, combined with a gentle invitation to let go and open, or breathing while calling in any positive energy can interrupt the tendency to contract around fearful, worried or angry thoughts. When we breathe consciously our minds open and our bodies soften. We can embrace a very different sense of ourselves. When we can relax, become still and experience calm inside, powerful experiences can take place in the space or moments between the thoughts.

Affirmations, Mantras and Sounds of the Chakras

Words hold a vibration and Sanskrit is one of the oldest known languages on the planet. It is a vibrational language. This is why the use of mantras can be so powerful. Like affirmations mantras are creating positive messages and vibrations. Both mantras and affirmations can be repeated while resting in restorative postures to cultivate a loving vibration within the practitioner.

I recommend Louise Hay's *Heal Your Body* as a wonderful resource for affirmations; it is also available in Spanish as *Sana tu Cuerpo*. For a deeper understanding of mantras I recommend Thomas Ashley-Ferrand's book, *Healing Mantras*.

While resting in the restorative asanas you can chant the Bija or Seed Mantras and visualize the colors of one or each of the chakras. Chant from 1st to 7th chakra focusing for 30 seconds to 1 minute on each chakra. Focus on the chakra as you chant the sound.

Chakra	Bija Mantra	Vowel Sound	Color	Function
1	Lam	o	red	security, survival
2	Vam	oo	orange	sexuality, emotions
3	Ram	ah	yellow	power, will
4	Yam	ay	green	love, relationships
5	Ham	ee	indigo	creativity, communication
6	Om	mm	purple	intuition, witness consciousness
7	Silence	ng	violet	awareness, understanding

Prayer

"When you pray from your heart you will know the truth and the truth is the answer to your prayers." Grandma Victoria Chipps, Lakota Elder

I spent a number of years with a Native American Medicine Family assisting and participating in their sacred and beautiful ceremonies, all of which were prayer based. Prayer is another powerful way to shift the focus from the mind to the heart, connect profoundly inside and receive guidance from your deepest self, spirit, god or goddess. Prayer is an opportunity to express what is in your heart and can be used to seek guidance, gain understanding, receive love, support and connection. Prayer is practiced in many traditions around the world and can be incorporated into the restorative practice. This can be done while you are in a restorative position or at the beginning or end of your practice.

Gratitude

This simple and powerful practice can shift your energy and moment quite quickly. Think of what you are grateful for, be it a person, an animal, an event. Think of one or many things. This can be practiced in meditation in any asana anywhere anytime--another example of using thought to shift vibration. An attitude of gratitude is a method that is practiced in many spiritual traditions.

Visualizations

There are countless healing visualizations that can be used with your resting poses. When leading visualizations make sure your voice is coming from an authentic and relaxed place. While you lead the visualization bring yourself there too so you enter into the relaxed and special place with your students. The effects of visualization have been proven to be more powerful when practiced from a relaxed state. You can use progressive relaxation in any of your resting poses. Here are a few examples of visualizations you can use after your students are relaxed. There are also a few others included with the posture explanations:

Find Yourself Someplace in Nature: After moving through a progressive relaxation and with your student(s) in a relaxed state, have them imagine themselves somewhere in nature, be it in the mountains, by a lake or ocean, in a forest, or on a hilltop or in a field. It may be someplace you have been or it may be someplace imagined. Engage as many senses as you can, seeing the details of your surroundings, smelling the air, noticing if you are alone or if someone is with you. Feel the air touch your skin--is it dry or moist; are there birds or animals nearby; is it windy or still? Once you can see and feel your surroundings drink in the healing energy of the natural world that surrounds you, drink in the tranquility and peace that is waiting for you and take it into your being and relax in this safe and healing space.

Ocean Waves: Notice your breath. Watch how your body rises and falls to receive and release the breath. Imagine your breath like a wave washing over you. As you inhale the wave comes up and washes over you, as you exhale the wave draws out any dis-ease or distress and takes it back to the sea. Inhale and the wave washes over you; as you exhale the healing waters enter into your cells and carry away any toxins or disharmony. Continue to see this for four breaths in and out. You can repeat this or embellish it as you like.

Healing Colors Surround You: Imagine a color that feels healing to you and begin to see and feel that color surrounding you. Imagine you could breathe that color into your body and begin to fill your body with your color with each inhalation. With each exhalation imagine the color spreading throughout your body. If there is an area of your body that is in need of more attention see the color filling that area, swirling and healing it with its vibrational rays of colorful light. Rest absorbed in this healing color and feel yourself being soothed and stress melting away. (Allow your student(s) to rest for a few minutes here with their healing color surrounding them.)

Love for a Small Baby or Child: Imagine yourself holding an infant or a small child. See and feel the innocence of this little being. Feel the love you have for them, pure and unconditional. Now direct the same loving energy towards yourself and allow yourself to be filled with this nurturing loving kindness.

Receiving a Loving Message: Once you or your student(s) are in a relaxed state you can visualize either an angel, a person who is special to you or a box on a table or on an altar. The message will come on a piece of paper, or it may be given directly in words. Receive the message from this being, person or place. Take it into your heart. Keep it with you. You may write it down when you finish the session.

Calling in Different Energies

You can call in different energies as a teacher to support your teaching, and you can also facilitate your students in calling in energies to support their restorative practice. Some possible energies to call in: relaxation, loving kindness, compassion, patience and gentleness. Remember, these energies already exist. They don't need to be created; they just need a sincere invitation. Calling in different energies is like tuning into a different radio station. Each station has a frequency, so you are tuning into a different frequency with the help of your mind and your consciousness.

Simply ask and surrender. For example: I call in the energy of love. I ask that the room be filled with loving energy. May each student be surrounded by loving energy. See, feel and know it to be true, then notice what happens. Make yourself a conduit. Allow yourself to become like empty bones so positive energies can flow through you.

Music versus Silence

This is a personal decision. Music can affect the students in your class to different degrees depending on the music and on the students. Music is also a vibrational frequency. This frequency will affect your students. If you choose to use it, make sure you, as the teacher or as a practitioner, always resonate with the music you have selected. That way it is more likely to assist and enhance your teaching, and it doesn't become a distraction for you (or for your students). Silence is also very powerful. It can leave an open space for the reality of what is in the moment. Sometimes a combination of music and silence can make sense.

Helpful Words

The following are helpful words or phrases to use while students are resting in their restorative asanas:
- Receive yourself as you are, drop any expectations, make space for all of who you are in this moment.
- Go inside and give yourself the gift of your own presence.
- Listen to your breath, feel yourself in this moment.
- Become present with yourself, nothing more, nothing less.
- For the next few minutes you have nothing to do, no place to go, just rest.
- Hold yourself gently as you rest.
- Do absolutely nothing.
- Relax everything.
- Leave your worries at the door. You can pick them back up as you leave if you choose to do so.
- Cultivate an attitude of kindness.
- Cultivate an attitude of compassion.
- Cultivate an attitude of_____(you fill in the blank).

Make a list of your favorites.

CHAPTER 8

Pranayama, Yogic Breath

"As long as there is breath in the body there is life. When breath departs, so too does life. Therefore regulate the breath."
Hatha Yoga Pradipika - Ch.2:S.3

There are many pranayama or yogic breathing techniques. Pranayama helps to still the mind and revitalize the body. I recommend these to be integrated with the poses or in seated meditation as part of a restorative practice. Other pranayamas can be integrated into the practice also.

Full Yogic Breath

This is a three-part breath. The breath can be soft yet enter all the torso. Breathe all the way down to the floor of the pelvis and then up into the abdomen, expanding the rib cage and into the chest. Breathe into the front, back and sides of the body. Exhale from the top of the chest down to the floor of the pelvis. The three parts of the breath are the lower abdomen, the rib cage and the chest. These parts can be broken down and practiced separately and then practiced all together.

Some of the Benefits
Calms the body and mind
Supports the digestive system
Massages the abdominal organs
Massages the lymph system
Opens and helps the rib cage and sternum area to open
Supports the respiratory system
Lowers blood pressure

Ujjayi Breath

Sometimes called the Ocean Sounding Breath. Imagine you are fogging up a mirror and breathe out of the mouth with a slight constriction in the back of the throat. Now breath in through the mouth with the same constriction. Close your mouth, keeping the constriction in the back of the throat as you breath in and out. Listen for the sound of the waves rolling in and out as you inhale and exhale through the nose. Allow the exhalation to be up to twice as long as the inhalation.

Some of the Benefits
Calms the mind
Supports the immune system
Reduces stress
Strengthens the nervous system

Nadi Shodana with Breath

Using your right hand, close off the right nostril with the thumb.
Breathe in through the left nostril, close both nostrils (using the ring finger or index finger); then lift the thumb to open the right nostril and breathe out though the right side. Breathe in through the right nostril, close both nostrils and release left side and breathe out through the left nostril. This completes one cycle.

Some of the Benefits
Lowers heart rate
Reduces stress and anxiety
Balances the left and right sides of the brain
Cultivates clear thinking

Nadi Shodana Energetically

This breathing variation was taught to me by a dear friend; she learned it from her Ayurveda teacher and I have found it to be quite powerful. Imagine the energy coming up from the earth through the left side of your body as you inhale into the left nostril and left side of the body without physically closing the nostril. Imagine exhaling down and out of the right side of the body and back in to the earth. Imagine inhaling up through the right side and nostril of the body and imagine breathing out the left nostril and left side of the body. Imagine breathing in through the left side again and imagine breathing out through the right nostril and side of the body. See a circuit of energy that moves from down in the earth and up into the heavens or at least up over the top of the head and back down again.

CHAPTER 9

Addressing Different Types of Students

"There is no remedy for love but to love more."

Henry David Thoreau

Before I address the postures I want to address a few types of students that I have met with in my years of teaching and how to support them and your class.

The healthy, active, connected student: These are students who know their bodies, understand how to use the props and are able to move in and out of many asanas. Use them as a model to help the class run smoothly, especially if you have newer students attending. Be sure to look for and help them with their alignment if needed or a supportive assist. Sometimes the best students can get overlooked.

The student with an illness or recovering from an illness: This student may need some extra loving care. Be sure they know they can go as slowly as they need to. Find out what is their illness and what they can and cannot do before class. Allow them to educate you about their situation if you are not familiar with it. If you or they are not sure about what is appropriate ask them to check with their doctor. (The Internet is a great resource to help to educate you about a specific illness. Don't be afraid to do your own research after class.)

The student who needs extra assistance for physical reasons: When there are students that need extra help assess the general needs of the class and decide who you will assist first so that all can be attended to in a quick and orderly fashion. Sometimes I go back and forth between students. You can help the ones who might not need too much assistance first and then move onto the ones who need more attention.

The student who cannot figure out how to use the props: Be patient and be willing to show them as many times as it takes. Help them to feel comfortable not remembering and eventually they will.

The stressed-out student: Keep inviting them to breathe and relax. Your touch can also be helpful to help them to reconnect with their bodies and breathe. If you are not familiar with the student always ask permission before touching them or until you get to know them better.

The emotional student: Be sure to have Kleenex handy in all your classes for noses and tears. Tears are invited to class and can be a wonderful release for students. Offer support at the end of class if this student wishes to share with you.

The student with an injury: Understand their injury and what they can and cannot do. Ask them if you aren't sure. Help them with variations to allow them to feel at ease and comfortable.

The student with anxiety: Work with the breath and address the mind. There are often conscious and unconscious physical tensions held in the body that can be focused on. Check for shoulder tension and constriction around the chest. Using a combination of words, postures and other techniques offered in this manual this student can gain enormous benefits from this practice.

The student with any one of a variety of physical conditions: These conditions can include but are not limited to low back issues, sciatica, knee, ankle, shoulder, neck, hip or foot issues. These are addressed with each posture in Chapter 10 under variations for different concerns.

See Chapter 12 for working with students with specific conditions.

CHAPTER 10

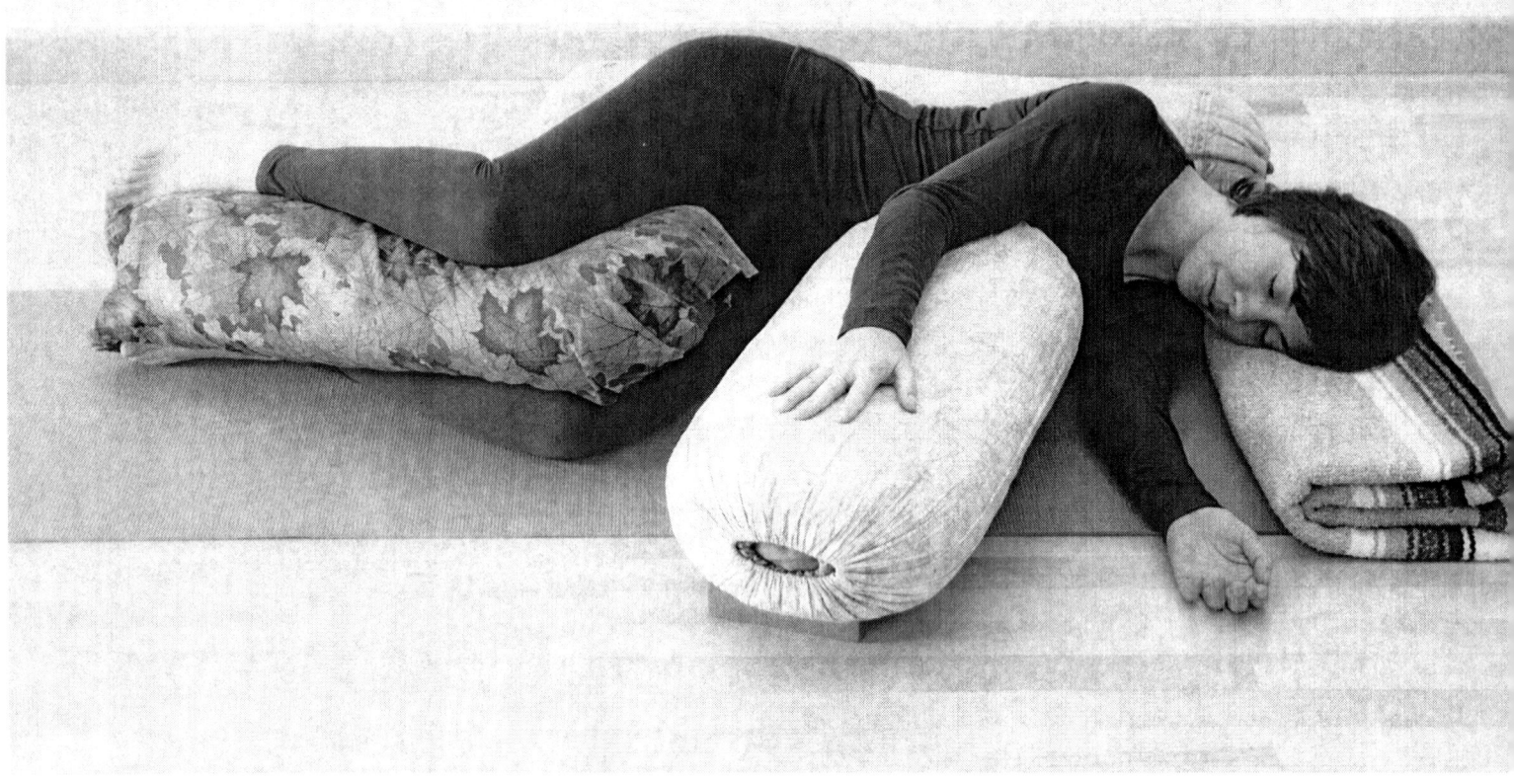

Restorative Asanas (Postures) in Detail

"How beautiful it is to do nothing, and then to rest afterward."

Spanish proverb

Below is the format in which each restorative pose is described. Use this as a guide to more fully understand each pose. For each restorative posture there is a basic position that has a variety of alternative possibilities, depending on the individual needs of your students.

Translation Here you will be provided with the translation from Sanskrit to English of each pose. Sometimes this can give you more insight into the posture and an understanding of the Sanskrit language.

General Overview This is where general information about each pose is given.

Basic Props Needed This section will describe the basic props needed for the pose. This is always subject to change depending on the needs of your students. Also be prepared to think outside the box with prop use. Many household items can be used as props such as phone books, couch cushions, folded sheets, towels or blankets. Sometimes you may discover just the right prop for a particular student that may work for their individual situation (see page 28). As students rest and begin to relax their body temperature drops so it is helpful to have a blanket available if needed.

Getting In and Out Each pose has a standard way to move in and out of the posture. Sometimes these need to be adjusted for individual students' needs.

Variations for Different Concerns There are always variations or another posture that can be used to address specific conditions. Here common themes and variations will be given for each position. All the major joints including ankles, knees, hips, sacrum, spine, shoulders, elbows, wrists, hands, and any muscular problems may be addressed here. This may also include variations for pregnancy.
In all the poses the posture should feel supported, steady and comfortable.

Therapeutic Applications Each pose may have one or more therapeutic applications that will be listed here.

Breath in Pose Breathing consciously while relaxing in the pose supports release in muscles and internal organs. It also stimulates the lymph system. Here cues about where to focus the breath and suggestions for how to breathe will be presented.

Verbal Cues There may be verbal cues and teachings to support your students in the asana. These are suggestions to help deepen the experience in the pose. They may be points of focus for the position or they may be visualizations or a meditative focus. These are a kind of assist that can be taken in through the mind and in some cases applied to the body or may address other states or levels of consciousness.

What to Look for With Alignment Every pose can be looked at with an eye for detail and balance. If a student lies back on a bolster and the bolster is crooked, then that will affect their body in the pose. When one side of the body is supported, the other side should also be supported. For example, in Supta Baddha Konasana (Reclining Bound Angle Pose), if one knee is supported because of hip or knee pain, the other side should also be supported so that an imbalance is not created.

Hands-on Assists Make sure that everyone is comfortable in the pose (including variations). This can keep you very busy depending on who is in the class and their level of experience with the postures.

Hands-on assists can be extremely important. Here you will be offered hands-on assist possibilities for each pose.

Take care of your body while assisting your students. Make sure as you assist you are not taxing your body. Keep your back straight, and squat, sit or pivot at the hips to keep your body happy and healthy. If you are sitting make sure you have support under your pelvis if needed.

Depending on the size of your class or if you are giving a private session, the amount of assists and time spent with each person will vary.

Refer back to Chapter 6 for more detailed descriptions of hands-on adjustments.

Pregnancy I have included a few words about variations for pregnancy but see Chapter 11 for more complete information.

How Long to Hold the Pose There will be a suggestion for each position as to the amount of time to stay resting in the position. Use your discretion.

Benefits Each posture has a variety of benefits listed for each position.

Contraindications Each posture has different contraindications or cautions – reasons or times to not practice the pose. Each posture will include an explanation of these.

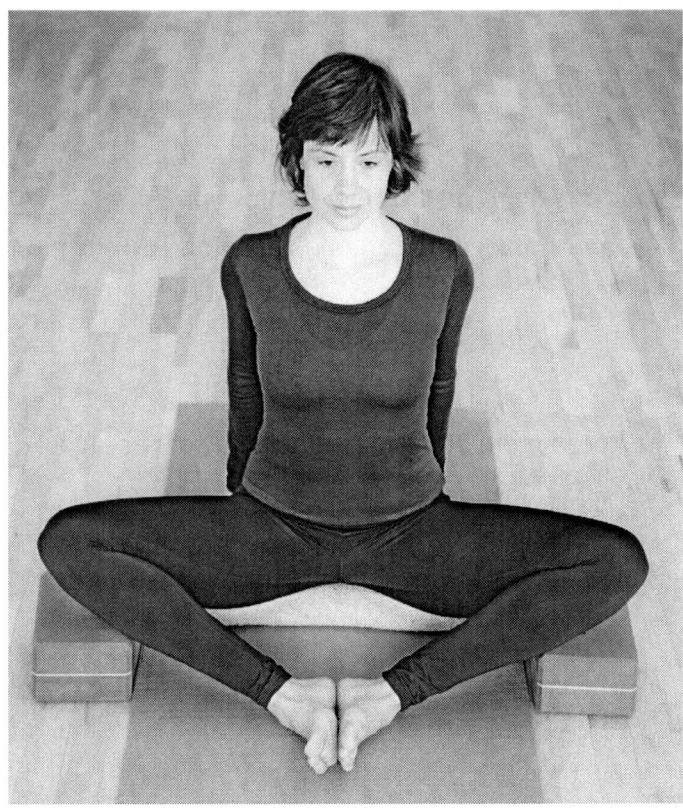

The Asanas

Supported Baddha Konasana (Supported Cobbler's Pose)

Seated and Forward Bends

Translation
Baddha means "fixed" or "bound" and kona means "angle."

General Overview
Sometimes called the butterfly pose, this is a great hip and groin opener. This was the position that cobblers in India used to work on the shoes they were fixing. They would put the shoe between their feet and hammer away.

Basic Props Needed
Two blocks or blankets and a folded blanket or pillow to support the sitting bones. For some students a wall may be needed to support the back.

Getting In and Out
Sit on the edge of your folded blanket. Bring the soles of your feet together evenly from toe to ball. Rest your knees on folded blankets, blocks or a combination of them. The height of the support is determined by the openness of your inner

Benefits

Helps relieve stiffness in the pelvic area

Opens the groins, inner thighs and knees

Stimulates the heart, ovaries and prostate gland, bladder, abdominal organs, and kidneys

Improves overall circulation

Relieves fatigue, anxiety and mild depression

Soothes sciatica

Alleviates menstrual discomfort

---

thighs. Support yourself with your fingertips on the floor behind you.

To come out straighten the legs on an outgoing breath. Transition to your next pose.

Variations for Different Concerns

Knee problems: try elevating the knees more or decrease the angle of the legs.

Back problems: elevate the pelvis, sit against a wall if needed.

Therapeutic Application

Sciatica

Tight hips

Asthma

Blood pressure

Flat feet

Infertility

Breath in Pose

Breathe normally through the nose.

Verbal Cues

Extend the spine.

Hold the ankles and extend upward.

Press the knees down into your support, then relax.

Place your hands on the knees, press down while trying to push the knees towards each other, then relax.

Press the outside edge of your feet together and press the big toenails outward and toward the floor as if you were opening the feet like a book.

Externally rotate the thighs.

What to Look for With Alignment

Feet are even from toe to heel.

If one knee is supported the other also needs to be supported.

The pelvis is upright.

The back is straight.

Hands-on Assists

Root the hips by pressing down on the legs as you move your hands to externally rotate the thigh, lengthening it from the hip creases out towards the knees.

Stand or kneel behind your student and gently pull their shoulder blades in and down the back.

Massage the shoulders with thumbs into the three points on tops of shoulders and/or gently knead the shoulders.

Manually open the feet.

Pregnancy

Regular practice throughout pregnancy can help ease labor and facilitate an easy delivery. (See p. 123 for more information about this posture during pregnancy.)

How Long to Hold the Pose

30 seconds to 3 minutes

Contraindications

In case of knee or groin injury, use a folded blanket for support under the thighs

Practice against the wall if student has asthma or bronchitis, breathlessness, rheumatoid arthritis or premenstrual stress

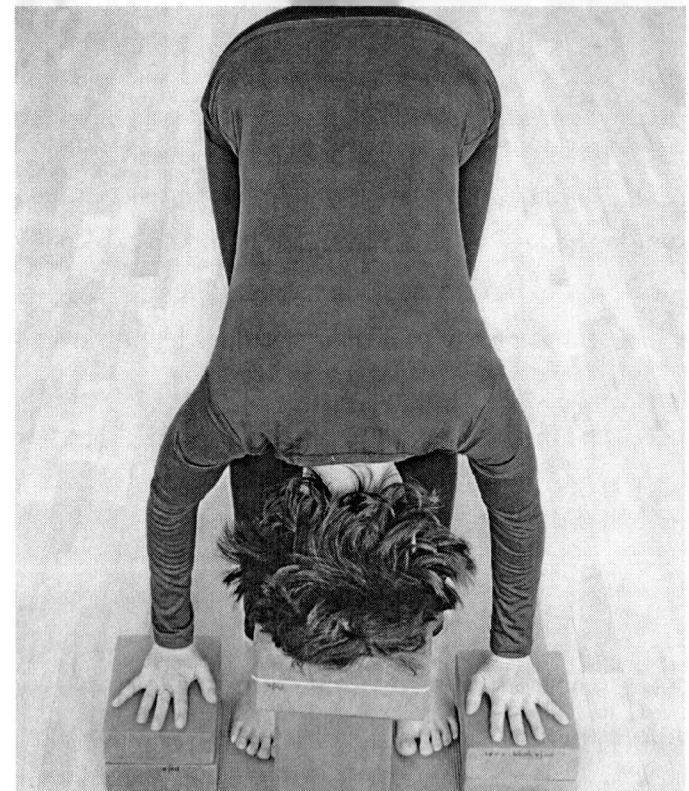

Benefits

Soothes and calms the body and nervous system

Reduces depression with regular practice

Reduces insomnia

Relieves fatigue

Increases blood flow to the brain

Regulates blood pressure

Tones abdominal organs

Strengthens and elongates hamstrings

Increases hip joint flexibility

Strengthens knee joint and surrounding tissue and muscle

Standing Supported Uttanasana (Standing Supported Forward Bend)

Translation
Ut means "deliberate" or "intense" and tana means "stretch," thus "intense forward stretch."

General Overview
This pose opens the back body while allowing support for the head and hands, creating a sense of relaxation permitting deeper opening in a forward bend. Little by little the body releases and fuller opening happens naturally.

Basic Props Needed
Several blocks, chair bolster combo

Getting In and Out
This asana can be done against the wall for additional support or in the center of the room. Stand with the feet parallel and hip width apart and play with the props to get a general idea of what will be needed. From standing position place the hands on the hips and extend upward, then keep extending as you lower down

and come to rest with the crown of the head just resting on the support so the neck is not constricted in any way and the hands come to rest flat on the block(s) and finger tips and toe tips are lined up evenly, if possible. If not, hands can come forward of the feet as necessary.

Variations for Different Concerns
If the legs are tight the head can rest on the seat of a chair with forearms or props on top of the seat.
Stack blocks for the hands so the palms are resting flat on the top of the blocks.

Therapeutic Applications
Depression
Blood pressure

Breath in Pose
Breathe normally

Verbal Cues
Soften the backs of the legs. Release the back of the neck. Allow the very top or crown of the head to gently rest on the prop.

What to Look for With Alignment
Check that the palms are flat on blocks. Use the widest part of the block if possible. Make sure the top of the head is resting on the block. As the body opens blocks can be removed.

Hands-on Assists
Neck release: Place your fingers very gently where the head meets the neck to bring the awareness to the neck while encouraging students orally to relax their neck. Gentle back and shoulder press to release holding.

Pregnancy
See p. 126 for more information about this pose in pregnancy.

How Long to Hold the Pose
15 seconds to 1 minute

Contraindications

Osteoarthritis of the knees

Diarrhea

Excessive curvature of the lumbar spine

Get up slowly if low blood pressure

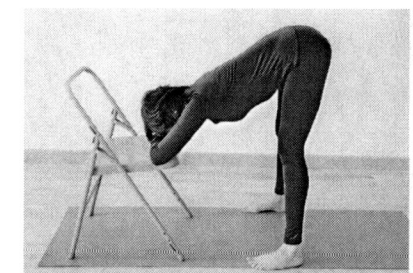

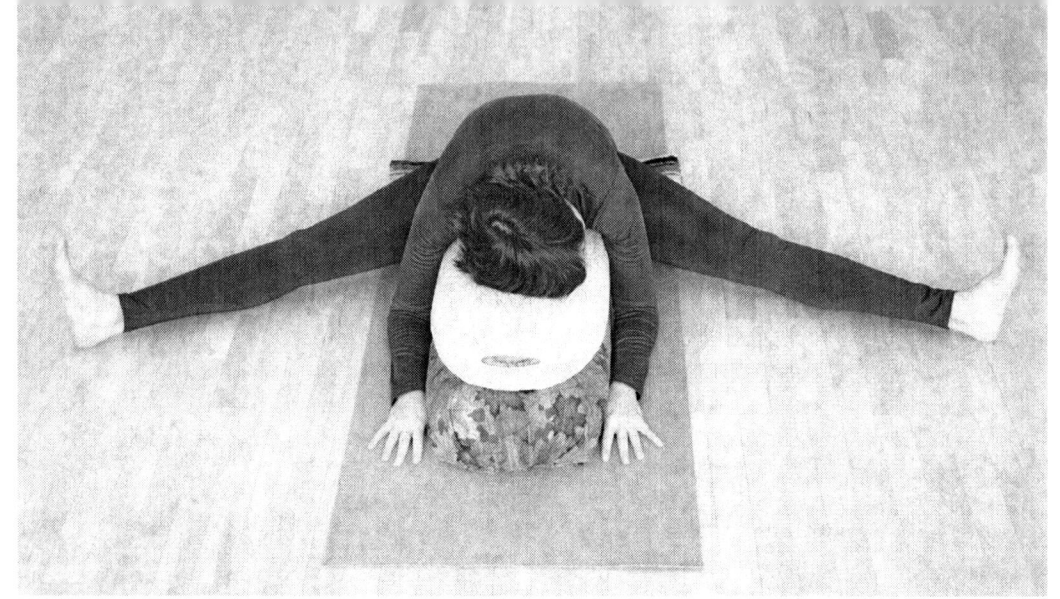

Supported Upavista Konasana
(Supported Seated Wide Angle)

Benefits

Helps with arthritis in the hip joints

Reduces or relieves sciatic pain

Helps prevent or relieve hernia

Massages reproductive organs

Benefits women during menstruation and pregnancy

Opens and releases hips

Opens groin muscles

Calms the brain

Translation

Upavista means "seated" and kona means "angle." Asana means "comfortable pose." Therefore Upavista Konasana means "Seated Wide Angle Pose."

General Overview

This is a wonderful posture that opens the legs and releases the pelvis and back. For students with tight hamstrings, tight back, tight hips or knee problems it can be challenging and may require many props.

Basic Props Needed

One or more bolsters plus blocks as needed and one or more folded blankets

Getting In

Sit on the edge of a folded blanket, open your legs wide out to the sides with your legs straight, press out through your heels with the tips of your toes facing the ceiling. Place your props in front of you and lean forward. Your whole body should be supported including the head. Stack as many or as few bolsters, blankets and blocks as needed. Press out through the heels stretching the legs, then relax. Breathe into the back of the body and the internal organs.

Getting Out
Place your hands under the shoulders and press up.

Variations
Low back discomfort: If the low back feels sore when leaning forward decrease the forward bend using more props under the front of the body to create less of an angle. Make sure the hips are elevated with a blanket or small pillow under the sitting bones; elevate higher if necessary. For some students a wall may be needed. If a student is unable to come forward at all they can work with elongating up the wall while grounding the pelvis. Support can be built up under their hands or forearms if possible.

Neck discomfort: The head can rest to the side, changing positions halfway through the hold time to balance the neck on both sides. If the neck is uncomfortable moving from side to side place a blanket or block under the forehead so that the neck is not turned and the face is looking towards the floor.

Inner thigh discomfort: If there is pain or strong pulling in the inner thighs bring the legs closer to each other; also make sure the pelvis is well supported.

Inner knee or back of knee discomfort: Try placing small cushions or rolled blankets under the knees, or if that does not help bring the legs closer together.

Breath in Pose
Breathe evenly; student can direct the breath into abdomen, low back or chest. Breathing consciously while relaxing in the pose supports release in muscles and internal organs. It also stimulates the lymph system.

Hands-on Assists
Massage shoulders.
Massage down the sides of the spine.
Press down on the thighs and depending on leg position roll thighs back or forward so that the toes are facing the sky.
From behind the student press the low back towards the floor placing the hands on with fingers facing the floor on either side of the low back.

Verbal Cues
Extend the spine as you move forward from the lumbar area.

Contraindications

Lower-back injury:
Sit up high on a folded blanket and keep your torso relatively upright

Use a chair if needed

Therapeutic Applications
Arthritis

Sciatica

What to Look for With Alignment
The pelvis is supported.
The back is straight and supported fully.

Pregnancy
The belly should never be crunched, and the spine always elongated. There should never be any pressure on the baby/belly. In the second and third trimester it can be practiced with the forearms on the seat of a chair to support the body elongating and moving forward only so much so the spine is long and the belly open with no pressure of any kind on the baby. (See p. 128 for more information about this posture during pregnancy.)

How Long to Hold the Pose
1 to 2 minutes

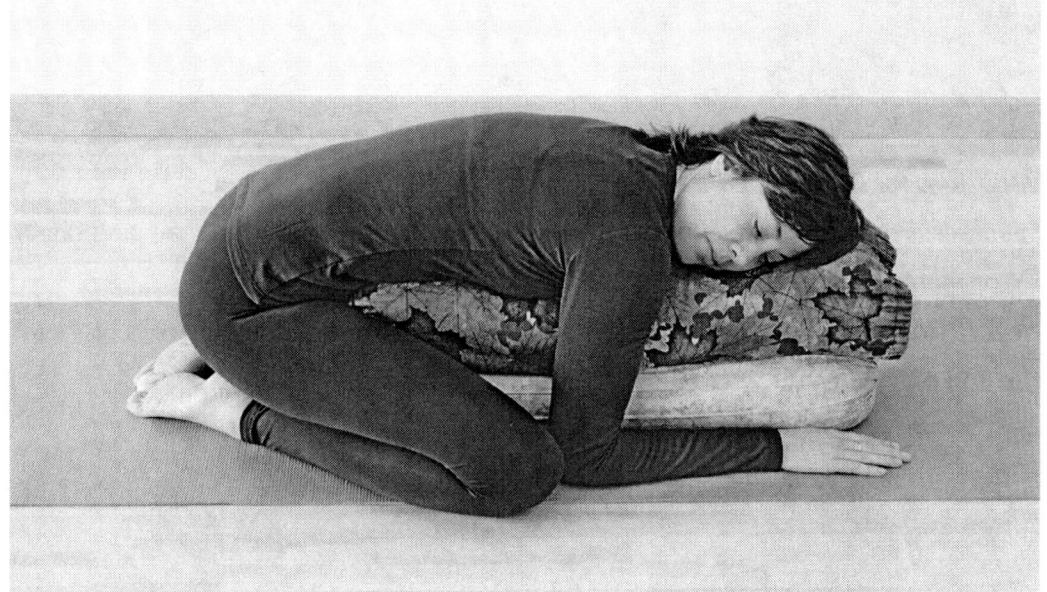

Balasana
(Supported Child's Pose)

Translation
Balasana means "pose of the child."

General Overview
This asana gives a feeling of support and security and is a great counter pose to Supta Baddha Konasana or other back bending asanas. It creates a massage for the internal abdominal organs and for the kidneys and adrenal glands when the breath is directed there.

Basic Props Needed
Bolster with two blocks below (will vary with size of your student) one at each end of the bolster or two bolsters one on top of the other.

Getting In and Out
Sit on the heels and open the knees. Pull the bolster and block set up between the legs. Place the hands on the thighs pressing down while extending the spine upward. Lay the torso over the bolster from pubic bone to the top of the head. Relax over the bolsters with the forearms resting flush to the floor and creating a right angle between the upper and lower arms.
To come out place the hands on either side of the bolster on the floor under the shoulders and press up.

Benefits

Gently opens the hips, thighs and ankles

Calms the brain

Relieves stress and fatigue

Massages internal organs

Relieves back pain

Relieves neck pain when practiced with variation, forehead on bolster

Variations for Different Concerns

Shoulder discomfort: Use support under the forearms, widen the arms and check for proper bolster height.

Neck Discomfort: The pose can be practiced with the forehead resting on a block off the end of the bolster with the legs extended outward.

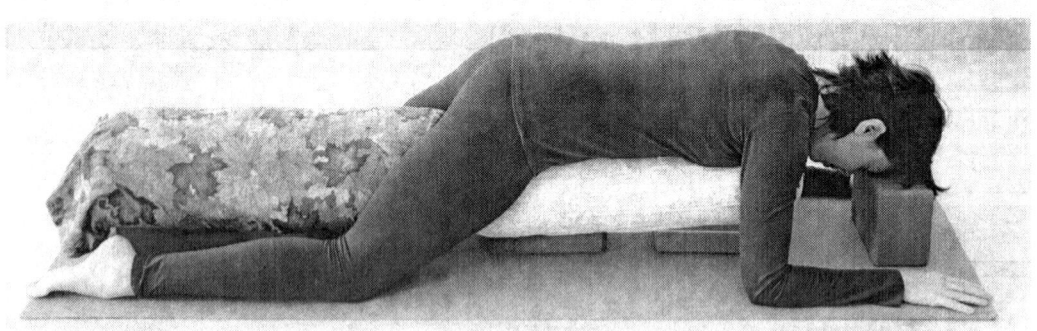

Knee discomfort: Place eye bags at the knee crease or use rolled-up towels or the like. If this does not relieve the discomfort use the legs extended version.

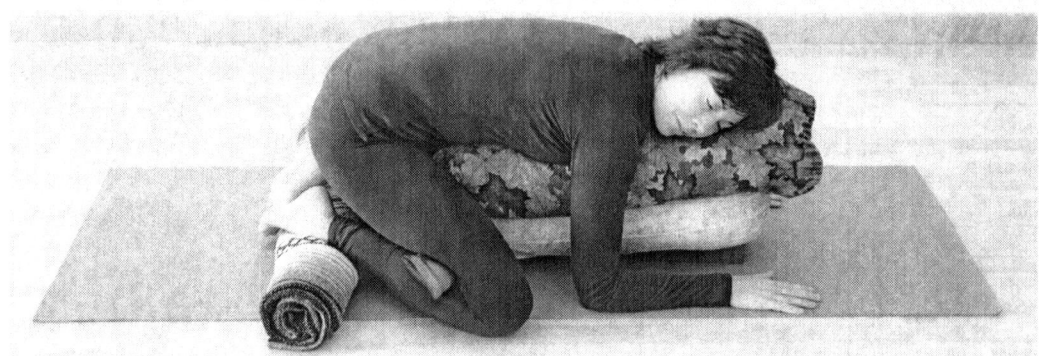

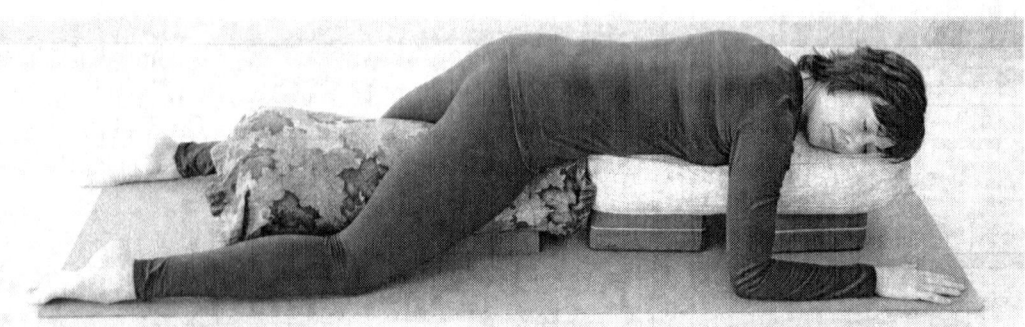

Ankle discomfort: Place something below the ankle to lift up the ankle away from the floor. If this does not relieve the discomfort use the legs extended version.

Foot discomfort: Same as for ankle.

If this does not relieve the discomfort use the legs extended version. The legs straddle the back bolster.

Therapeutic Applications

Stress relief

Breath in Pose

Breathe consciously into the low back, kidneys and adrenals. Breath can also be directed into the abdomen.

Verbal Cues

Direct the breath focus, and encourage the focus on feeling secure and innocent like a child.

What to Look for With Alignment

Big toes touching

Upper arm perpendicular to floor, forearms resting on the floor

Buttocks as close to heels as possible in the bent leg version

Hands-on Assists

Use the back press downward technique, pressing the hands on the back from sacrum to upper back on either side of the spine.
Use the diagonal low back press to stretch from shoulder to ilium on both sides.
Press hands into low back; use your body weight to press the pelvis away from the head and open the low back.
Massage on either side of the spine with thumbs or palms.
Massage shoulders.

Pregnancy

This pose can be practiced with the variation of bolster rests under the chest; baby rests between the bolster and the pelvis. Knees open wide. The bolster is primarily under the chest. (See p. 131 for more information about this posture during pregnancy.)

How Long to Hold the Pose

2 minutes to 7 minutes including neck to both sides

Contraindications

Diarrhea

Knee injury (variation with legs extended)

Ankle injury (variation with legs extended)

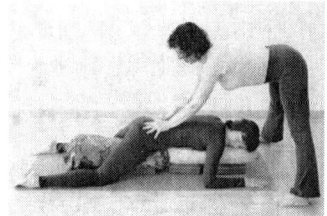

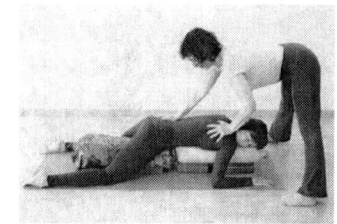

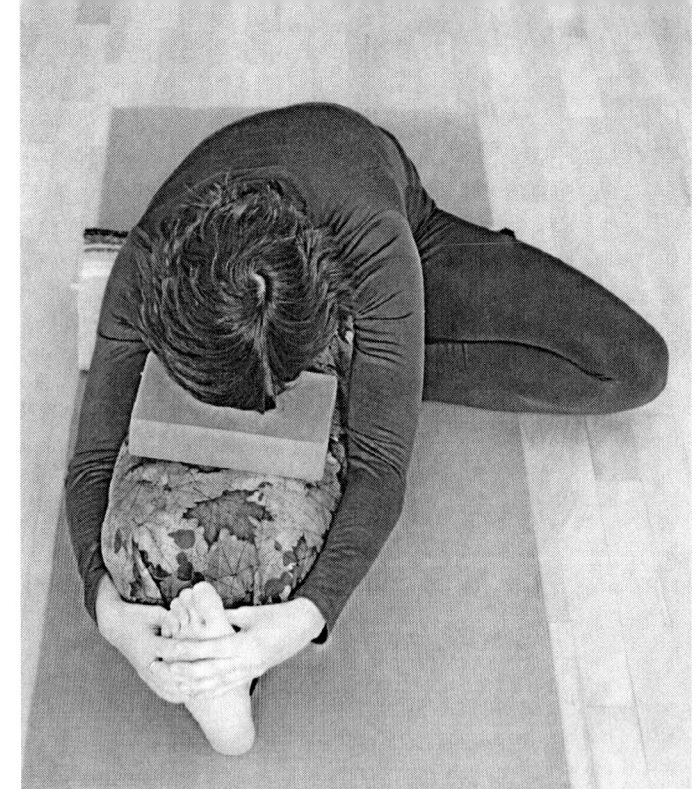

Benefits

Calms the mind and helps relieve mild depression

Stretches the spine, shoulders, hamstrings, and groins

Stimulates the liver and kidneys

Improves digestion

Normalizes blood pressure

Improves bladder control

Helps relieve the symptoms of menopause

Relieves anxiety, fatigue, headache, menstrual discomfort

Prevents fibroids and regulates menstrual flow

Supported Janu Sirsasana (Seated Angle Head to Knee)

Translation
Janu means "knee" and sirsa means "head." Hence it is the head to knee pose.

General Overview
This is a wonderful pose to relax the nervous system. It soothes irritability and restlessness of the mind. This is a calming posture.

Basic Props Needed
Folded blanket, bolster(s), block

Getting In and Out
Sit on the edge of a folded blanket. Bend one leg and rest the sole of the foot on the inside of the opposite thigh. Rest your props on the extended leg, turn the torso toward the extended leg, come forward and down to be totally supported.

Variations for Different Concerns
Can be practiced with the back against the wall.
If your student can't reach the foot they can use a tie.

For knee problems use support under extended knee and/or under the bent leg knee.

Therapeutic Applications
Stress
High blood pressure
Insomnia
Sinusitis

Contraindications
Asthma

Diarrhea

Acute knee injury

Breath in Pose
Breathe into both sides of the body fully and evenly, then normally. Breathe into the back of the legs.

Verbal Cues
Relax the shoulders, relax the face.

What to Look for With Alignment
Reach both arms evenly to support both sides of the back to open.

Hands-on Assists
Use the low back press at an angle technique: Stand or kneel behind the student facing their back. Place your hands against their lower back and pelvis. The hands should be turned so the fingers point towards the tailbone. The pressure isn't to push them deeper into the forward bend; rather, gentle pressure (parallel to the line of the back in a downward direction towards the tailbone in line with the spine) encourages the spine and tailbone to lengthen away from the torso; ground them toward the earth and release the back gently. Massage the shoulders. Encourage the body to rest over the bolster with as much of the front of the torso resting on the bolsters as possible. Adjust the student's body gently and encourage extension, moving hands along the spine from the pelvis to the shoulders.

Pregnancy
This pose can be practiced coming forward and resting the head on the back of the hands and the forearms on the seat of a chair and keeping the spine long. Always maintain plenty of space for your baby. (See p. 134 for more about this posture during pregnancy.)

How Long to Hold the Pose
1 to 3 minutes per side

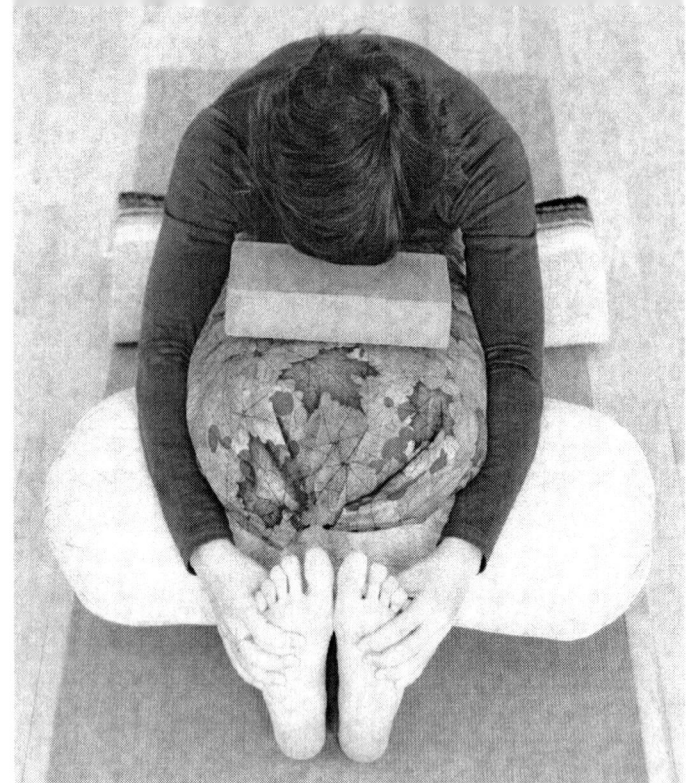

Benefits

Calms the mind

Relieves stress

Relieves mild depression

Stimulates the ovaries and uterus

Massages abdominal organs

Improves digestion

Reduces stress in facial muscles

Soothes headache

Soothes anxiety and fatigue

Supported Paschimottanasana, Forward Bend

Translation
Paschimottana means "intense stretch of the West." Pashima means "West," uttana means "intense stretch."

General Overview
This is a classic pose for opening hamstrings, releasing the back and opening the entire back side of the body.

Basic Props Needed
Blanket for under the pelvis; combination of bolsters, blocks and blankets

Getting In and Out
Students sit on the edge of a folded blanket. For students unable to sit without support for their backs, they can sit against the wall with support under their pelvis. Place a combination of props on the legs and rest forward so that the entire front body and head are supported. Rest the hands on the feet or use a tie.

Variations
Use a tie if feet are unavailable.
Place a blanket under the knees if student is unable to extend the legs completely.

Therapeutic Applications
Stress
Insomnia
High blood pressure
Infertility
Insomnia
Sinusitis

Breath in Pose
Breathing consciously while relaxing in the pose supports the release of muscles and internal organs. It also stimulates the lymph system.

Verbal Cues
Breathe into the backs of the legs and relax around the holding.

What to Look for With Alignment
Heels on the wall, forehead resting on a block, good for relieving cramps in the calf muscles, strengthening. Look for evenness in spine from pelvis to head and make sure the pelvis is supported.

Hands-on Assists
Work in partners to open the body first. Partner forward bend: One practitioner sits with legs crossed. The other extends the legs and the feet rest on the shins of the partner.

Use the low back press at an angle technique: Stand or kneel behind the student facing their back. Place your hands against their lower back and pelvis. The hands should be turned so the fingers point towards the tailbone. The pressure isn't to push them deeper into the forward bend; rather, gentle pressure (parallel to the line of the back in a downward direction towards the tailbone in line with the spine) encourages

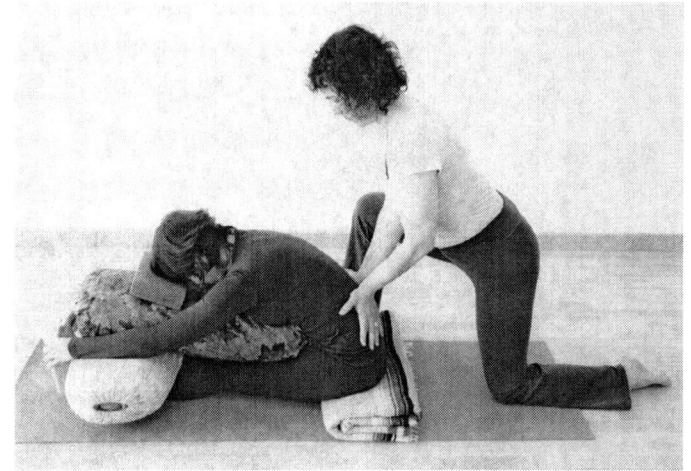

Sharpens memory

Soothes the sympathetic nervous system

Rests the heart

Cools the temperature of the skin

Relaxes the thyroid gland

Stretches the spine, shoulders, hamstrings and the entire back of the body

Helps relieve the symptoms of menopause and menstrual discomfort

Contraindications

Asthma

Diarrhea

Acute knee injury

the spine and tailbone to lengthen away from the torso; ground them and release the back gently.

Gently massage their shoulders and softly move down either side of the spine until you reach the low back.

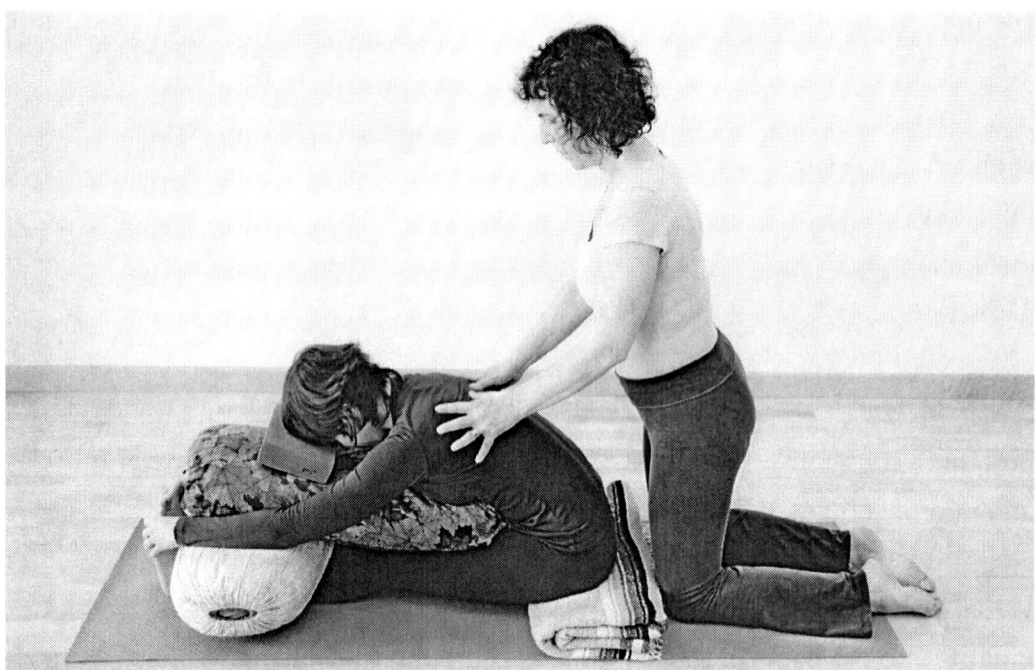

Pregnancy
Not to be practiced during pregnancy.

How Long to Hold the Pose
20 seconds to 5 minutes

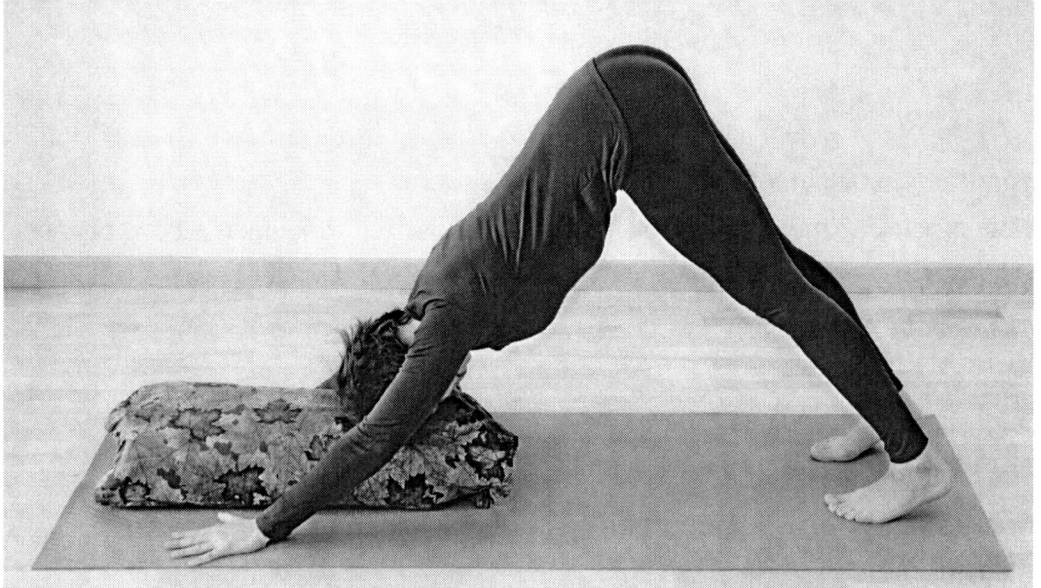

Adho Mukha Svanasana (Downward-Facing Dog)

Translation
Adho means "facing down" and Svan means "dog."

General Overview
This is the multivitamin asana of yoga that opens and strengthens the body; it is an excellent pose for opening the hamstrings, back, shoulders and hands while bringing strength to the arms, wrists, hands and torso.

Basic Props Needed
Mat, block(s) or bolster and a wall for three variations

Getting In
From Child's Pose extend the arms out on the floor, then plant the hands and come to table pose. Make sure the hands are well connected to the earth. The middle fingers are parallel, hands plugged into the earth like a plug into a socket, all the skin of the hand is touching the mat and the fingers are comfortably apart. Tuck the toes under and extend the legs till they are straight. Rest the forehead on a block or bolster.

Getting Out
To come out bend the legs at the knees and bring them to the mat.

Benefits

Calms the brain

Relieves stress

Relieves mild depression

Energizes the body

Opens the shoulders, hamstrings, calves, arches and hands

Strengthens the arms and legs and arches of the feet

Helps relieve the symptoms of menopause.

Relieves menstrual discomfort when done with head supported

Helps prevent osteoporosis

Improves digestion

Relieves headache

Alleviates insomnia

Reduces back pain

Alleviates fatigue

Variations for Different Concerns
Fingers going up the wall, head on block for arthritis or stiff shoulders, elbows or hands.

Therapeutic Applications
High blood pressure
Asthma
Flat feet
Sciatica
Sinusitis

Breath in Pose
Breathe normally through the nose.

Verbal Cues
Pull the thighs, knees and ankles back in the direction of the wall behind you. Press the hands completely into the floor. Rest the head and neck fully.

What to Look for With Alignment
When resting the head on a bolster or block be sure the student is not bending their arms to reach the block but opening the body enough with feet and hands away from each other to allow the forehead to reach the support.

Hands-on Assists

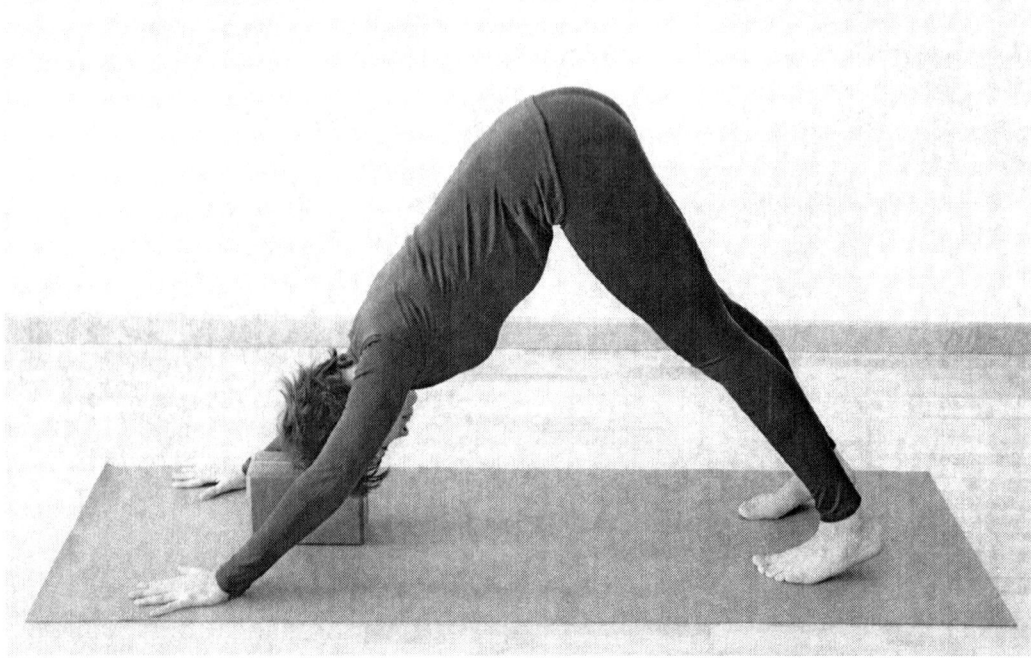

Put the tie around your student's low back and between their legs; stand behind the student and as if you were water skiing, pull up and back on the ends of the tie to release the pressure on the shoulders and arms and to encourage the internal rotation of the legs. This can be done with the head supported or not.
Press the low back pelvis area towards the coccyx.

Contraindications

Carpal tunnel syndrome

Diarrhea

Varicose veins

High blood pressure or headache: Support the head on a bolster or block

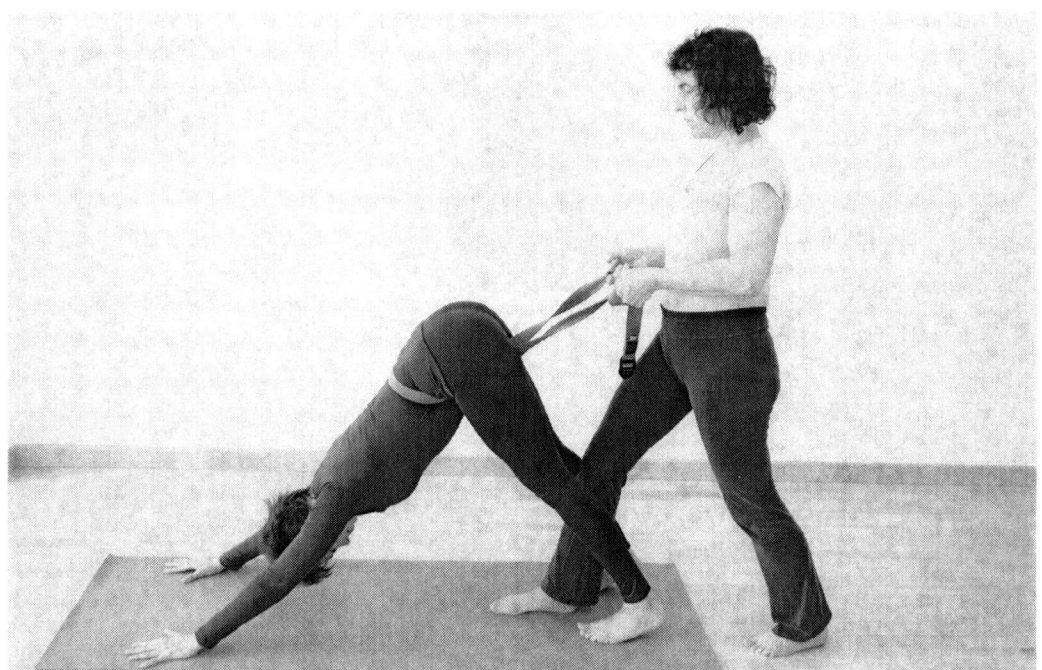

Pregnancy
Practice with shorter holding times especially at the end of the third trimester, as is comfortable (see p.137 for more information about this posture during pregnancy).

How Long to Hold the Pose
15 seconds to 1 minute

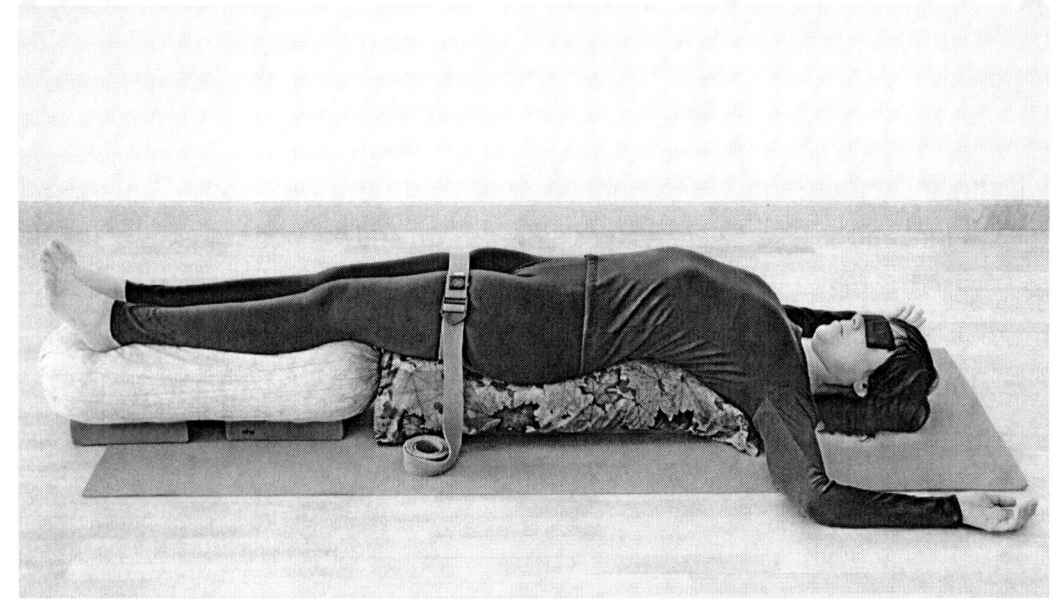

Back Bends

Setubandha Sarvangasana (Supported Bridge)

Benefits

Elongates the neck, spine and hips

Expands the chest

Improves circulation of blood

Translation
Setu means "bridge," bandha means "formation" and sarvanga means "entire body"; hence, the body forming a bridge.

General Overview
This is a deeply restful posture that helps to open the chest, revitalize the thyroid gland and calm the mind.

Basic Props Needed
A block, or two bolsters and block combo and a strap, or feet against the wall: one bolster, two or more blocks to support or elevate the feet and a strap

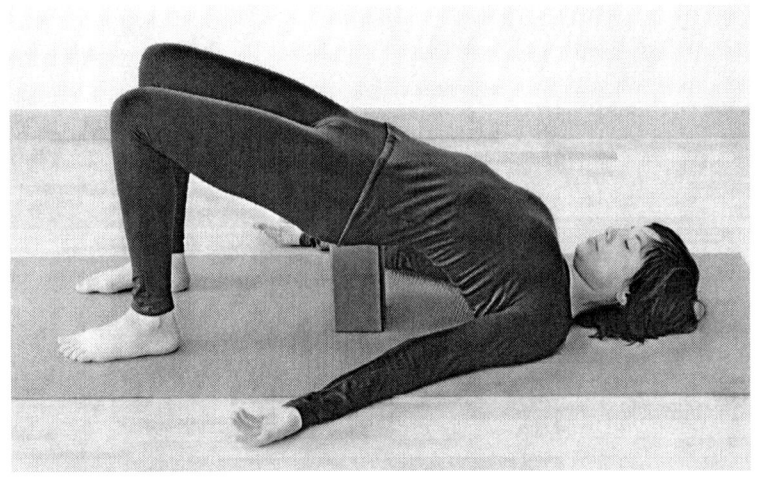

Getting In, Block Under Pelvis Variation
Lying on the back place the feet on the floor, lift the pelvis, slide block under sacrum, rest the sacrum onto the block. Use one of the three heights the block offers or a combination of blocks depending on the flexibility of the practitioner. To maintain the natural curve in the cervical spine and make sure there is space for the throat (and if you notice that space around the throat is needed), keep the chin slightly lifted.

Getting Out, Block Under Pelvis Variation
Press the feet into the floor, lift the pelvis and remove the block from under the pelvis. Slowly release to the floor, bring the knees into the chest.

Getting In, Bolster Variation
Lying on the back next to the bolster, measure along its side to where the bottom of the shoulder blades are even with the short end of the bolster. Keep track of where the buttocks are next to the bolster, and sit up and slide onto the bolster. Place the strap around the mid thighs; lie back. The tops of the shoulders should rest on the floor. Arms rest over head or to the sides.

Getting Out, Bolster Variation
place the feet on the floor, lift the pelvis up and either the student or the teacher slides the bolster out and places it under the knees lengthwise; drop the pelvis down and rest the knees over the bolster; rest for a few moments letting the back relax.

Variations
Low back discomfort: Adjust leg and feet position.
When practicing on bolsters or against the wall with the legs resting on blocks, raise the level of the legs further with bolsters and/or blocks.

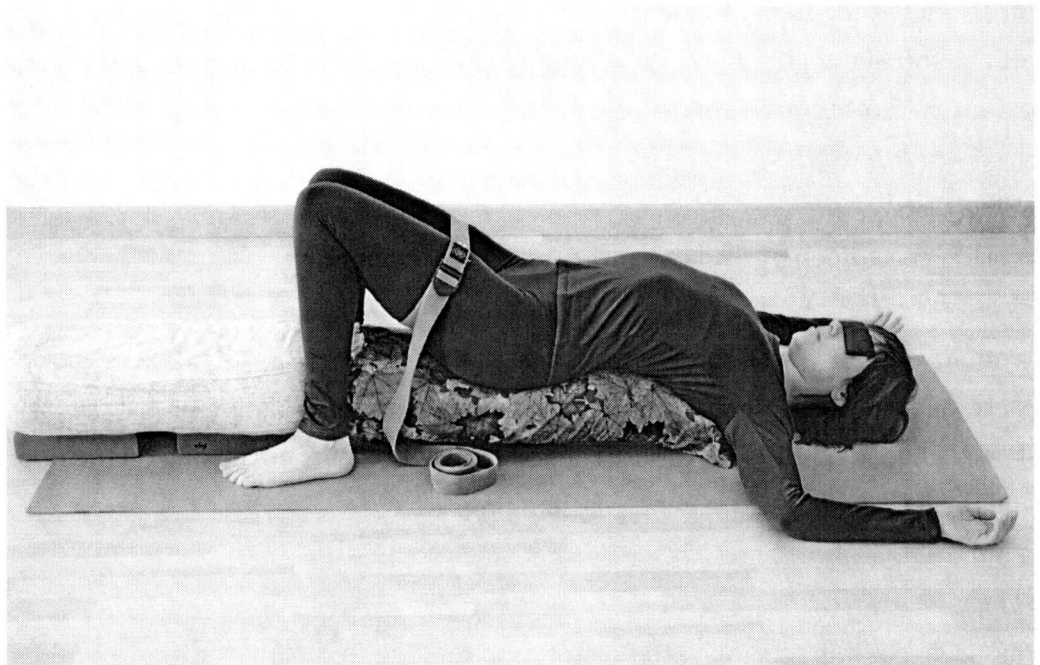

Helps alleviate stress and mild depression

Reduces fatigue, anxiety and insomnia

Calms the brain and central nervous system.

Improves digestion, strengthens abdominal organs

Helps relieve symptoms of menopause

Reduces backache and headache

Rejuvenates tired legs

Relieves symptoms of asthma

Can reduce high blood pressure

Prevents arterial blockages or heart attack by resting the heart and increasing blood circulation to the arteries

Stimulates the lungs, thyroid gland and abdominal organs

Prevents varicose veins

Contraindications

Low-back discomfort that cannot be relieved by variations

Shoulder discomfort: Adjust arm position.

Against the wall with one bolster and a block or blocks (this is a good variation if you don't have enough bolsters to use two per person).

Keep the legs together: Use a strap on the upper legs.

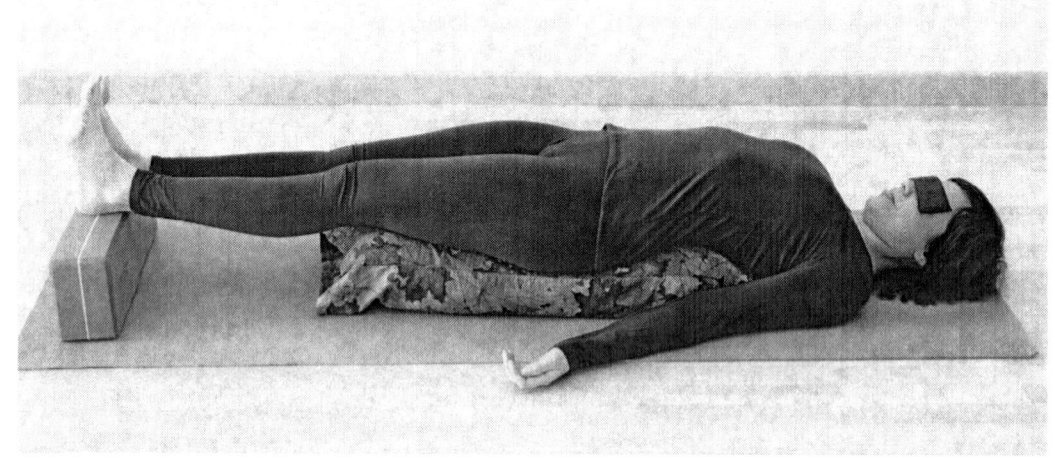

Therapeutic Applications
Hypertension
Sinusitis
Regulates blood pressure

Breath in Pose
Breath can be focused into the chest, rib cage and the front of the body. Breath can also be focused on the back body, into the kidney area and shoulder blades, elongating the back with the mind's eye then normal breathing.

Verbal Cues
Feel the chest opening and the entire front body elongating.

What to Look for With Alignment
Make sure the block is under the sacrum if practicing the variation with one block. If practicing on bolsters make sure the top of the shoulders are resting on the floor and the neck and head are in no way hanging.

Hands-on Assists
Massage feet if practicing with bolsters and feet are free. Note the blanket under the teacher's pelvis supporting her as she assists her student.

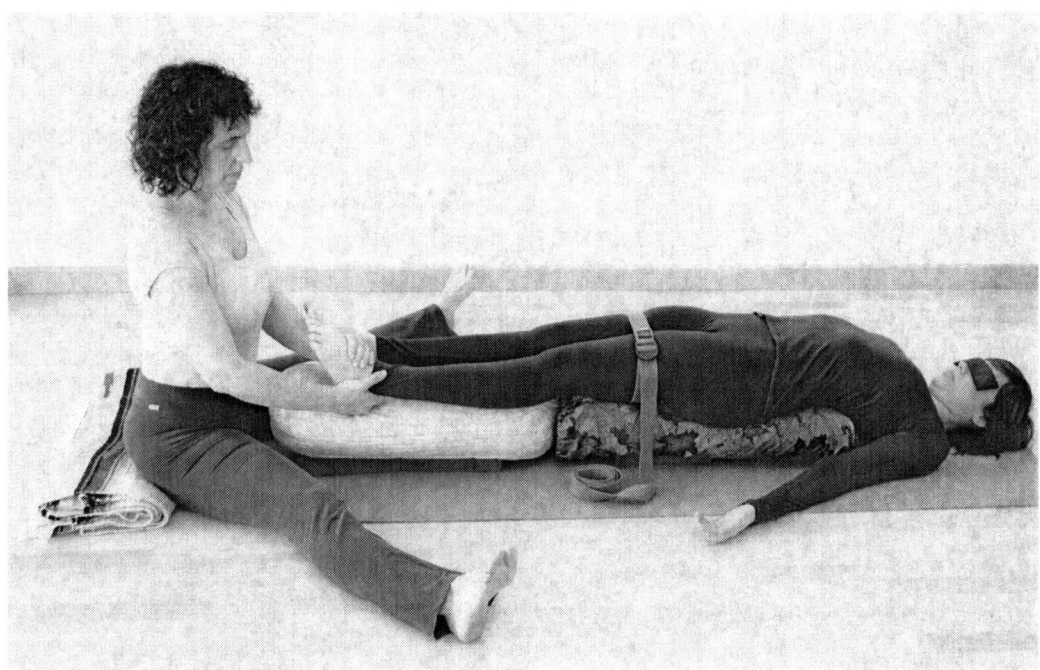

Sitting at the student's head gently lay the hands on the upper chest; or press finger tips or thumbs on chest points located just below the collarbones: Press thumbs starting at the center of the chest on either side of the sternum and press below the collarbone to stimulate the lung points, moving from the center outward.

Pregnancy
Do not practice after the first trimester.

How Long to Hold the Pose
3 to 10 minutes

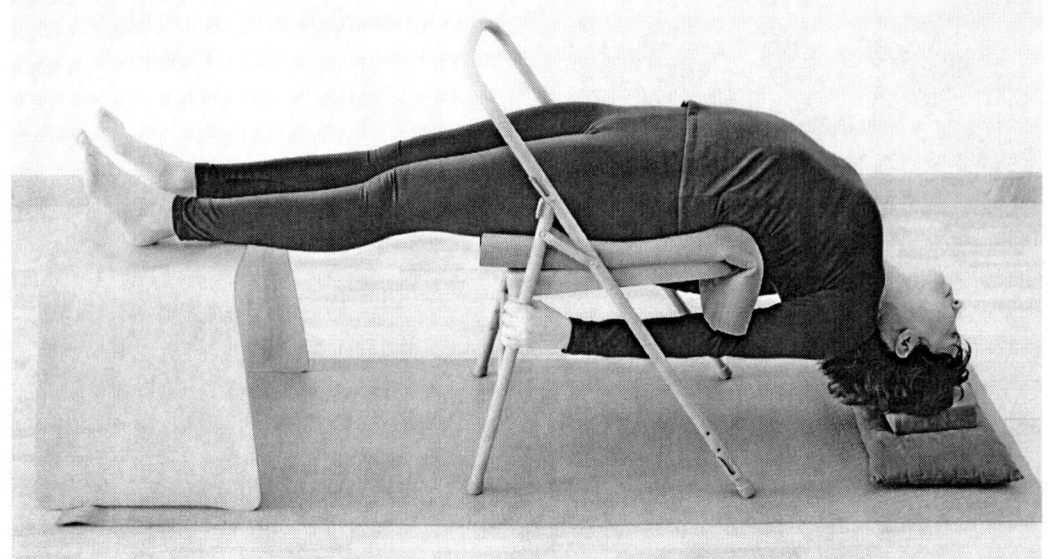

Benefits

Increases flexibility of the spine

Calms and quiets the mind

Soothing and relaxing to the brain

Increases lung capacity

Massages and strengthens the heart

Reduces menstrual and menopausal symptoms

Corrects displaced bladder or prolapsed uterus

Can relieve low back discomfort

Prevents varicose veins

Extends front of body

Tones internal organs

Stimulates the adrenal, thyroid, pituitary and pineal glands

Revitalizes central nervous system

Viparita Dandasana (Backbend with Chair)

Translation
Viparita means "inverted" or "reversed" and danda means "staff."

General Overview
This posture offers an intense back bend with support.

Basic Props Needed
Chair, yoga mat, block, bolster and/or several blankets, small towel.

Getting In
Fold up a mat and place it on the chair. Place a small towel on the chair to support the lower back. Sit and bring the legs through the chair sitting with back of the chair towards you and bring the legs together. If needed place a tie around the thighs if the legs splay apart. This is to help prevent the legs from rolling out and to prevent the compression in the low back. Lie back over the chair while holding on to the edge of the chair so that the edge of the chair is across the upper back beneath the bottom of the shoulder blades. Take hold of the back of the chair and slowly lower the head down then, either: a) bring the hands in between the front chair legs and take hold of the back legs of the chair, b) take hold of the elbows and extend the upper arms out alongside the ears, or c) extend the arms out and down towards the floor. Each of these arm positions gives the backward extension a different intensity. Extend the legs out as long as the back doesn't feel discomfort.

Getting Out

To come out of the pose, bend the knees and plant the feet on the floor. Bring the arms into the sides, and reach for the lower back of the chair. (If necessary, bring one hand to the head and lift the chin into the chest first.) Lift yourself up swiftly in one movement, keeping the head towards the chest. Sit in the chair with the arms resting on the chair back for a moment to allow the blood flow to equalize.

Variations for Different Concerns

If extending the legs or having the feet on the floor is too challenging for the lower back, stack the feet up higher, even to the extent of having a second chair or bench underneath them or put blocks under the feet.

Contraindications

Back injury

Stress-related headaches

Active migraine

Eye strain

Intestinal, constipation or diarrhea

Dizziness

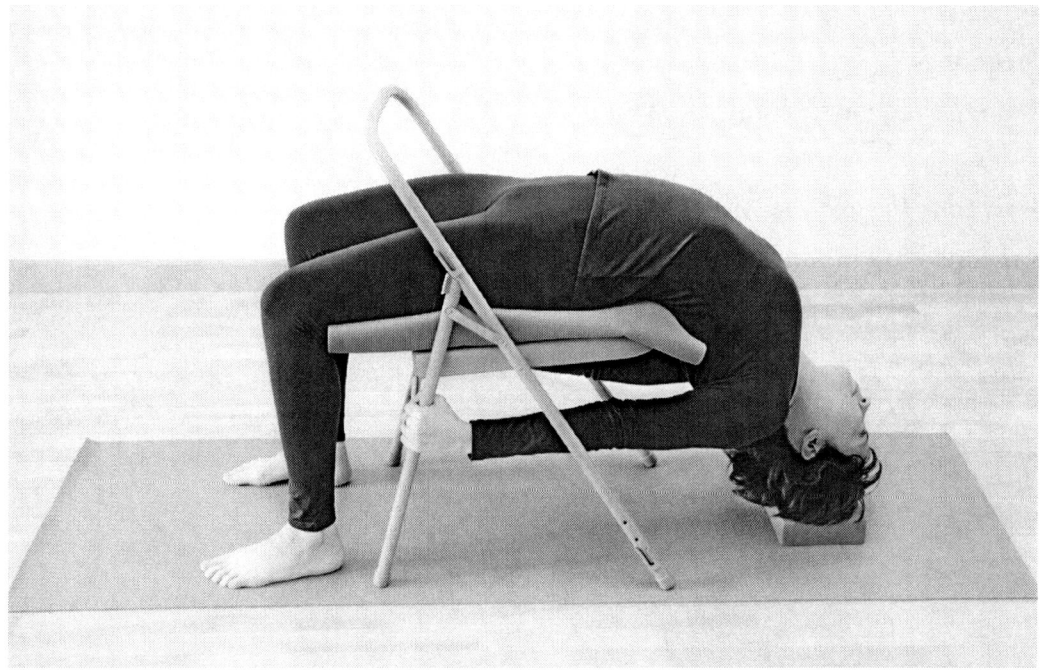

Therapeutic Applications

Depression

Low self esteem

Breath in Pose

Breathe fully into the chest and breath steadily and normally.

Verbal Cues

Roll the tailbone towards the heels and press the heels into the wall.
Stretch and lengthen the legs.

Broaden the back ribs.
Broaden the chest and collarbones.
Soften the neck.
Relax what doesn't need to be active.

What to Look for With Alignment
Make sure the head is supported without any pressure on the neck. Allow the top and/or the back of the head to be supported.

Hands-on Assists
When practitioner is coming out support the head as they come up.

Pregnancy
Not recommended during pregnancy.

How Long to Hold the Pose
5 seconds to 3 minutes

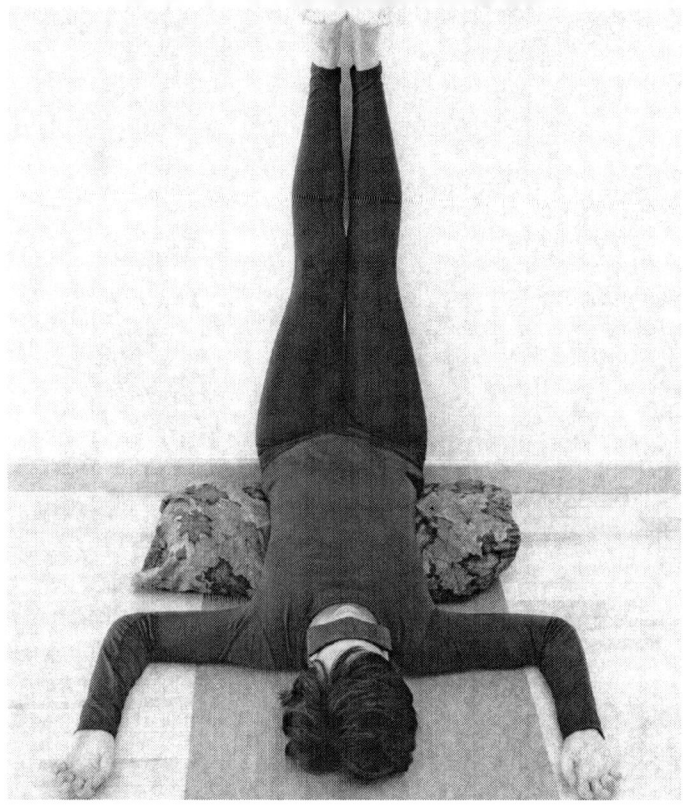

Viparita Karani (Legs up the Wall)

Inversions

Translation
Viparita karani means "inverted lake."

General Overview
This is a fantastic pose that has a few variations. It can be used as a passive inversion with the elevated version. It has many benefits that can be gleaned from practice.

Basic Props Needed
You will need a mat, blanket and, depending on your variation, a bolster.

Getting In and Out
The challenge of this pose can be getting into the pose. You want to get your buttocks as close to the wall as possible. When working flat you can lie down on your side with your buttocks touching the wall. This can be quite challenging for some students. Then swing the legs up the wall.
If you are practicing on a bolster, place the bolster a few inches from the wall so the bum can drop down into the space between the wall and the bolster. Sit with the

side of your body against the wall, on the edge of the bolster at one end with one buttock cheek on the bolster and the other in the air between the bolster and the wall; then swing the legs up the wall using your hands behind you to prevent you from moving away from the wall. Permit the buttocks to rest in the space between the bolster and wall; the belly should be parallel with the floor. To get out place the feet flat on the wall, lift the pelvis to slip out the bolster and release the pelvis to the floor; rest for a few breaths until the spine and the muscles of the back relax. Roll to one side and press up with the hands to seated position.

Variations for Different Concerns

On or off bolster: the asana can be practiced on the bolster or flat on the floor. Arm position can be changed if there are shoulder issues.

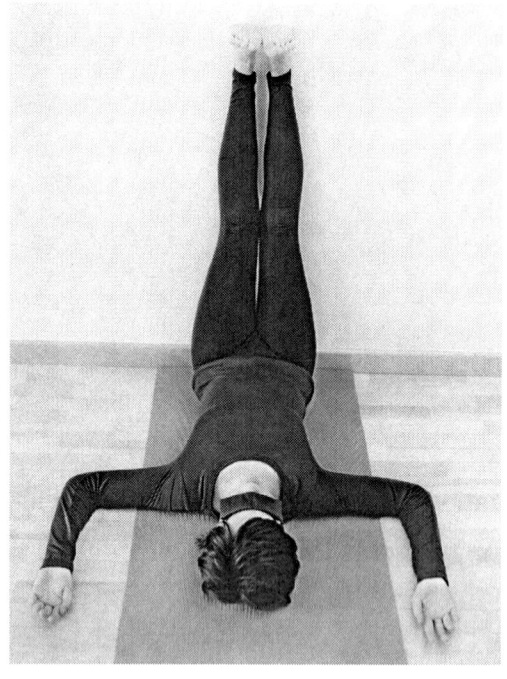
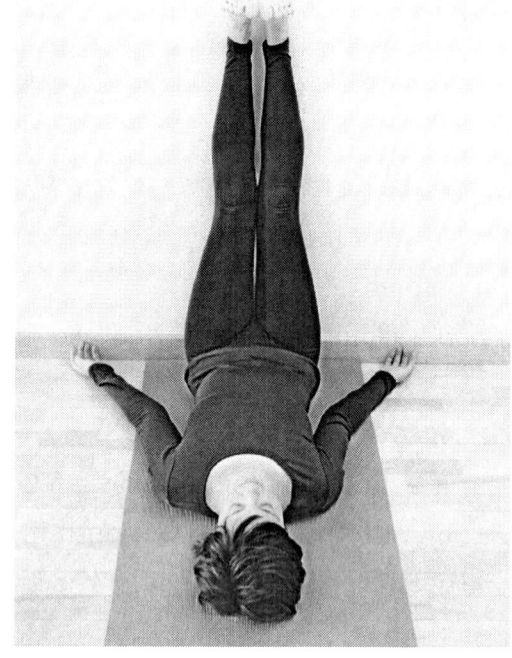

Leg variations: Upavista Konasana (open the legs into a "v" shape) and Baddha Konasana (place the legs in Cobbler's Pose on the wall) can both be practiced while resting directly on the floor or on a bolster. You can push your hands gently against the top inner thighs to stretch the groin.

With the legs straight up the wall you can place a loop in the strap around your thighs, just above the knees and tighten to hold the legs together, allowing relaxation in the legs and the groin to soften.

If flat on the floor you can also allow the legs to go to one side, sliding both legs along the wall to each side and taking a few breaths when in each direction. To

Benefits

Relieves anxiety

Relieves arthritis

Eases digestive problems

Relieves headaches

Regulates high and low blood pressure

Insomnia

Migraine

Mild depression

Respiratory ailments

Urinary disorders

Varicose veins

Menstrual cramps

Premenstrual syndrome

Menopause

come up, lead with the leg that is on top and allow the lower leg to follow naturally. Once in the pose, with the legs up the wall, back-flat-on-the-floor version, bend your knees and slide your feet down the wall. This can further release the back.

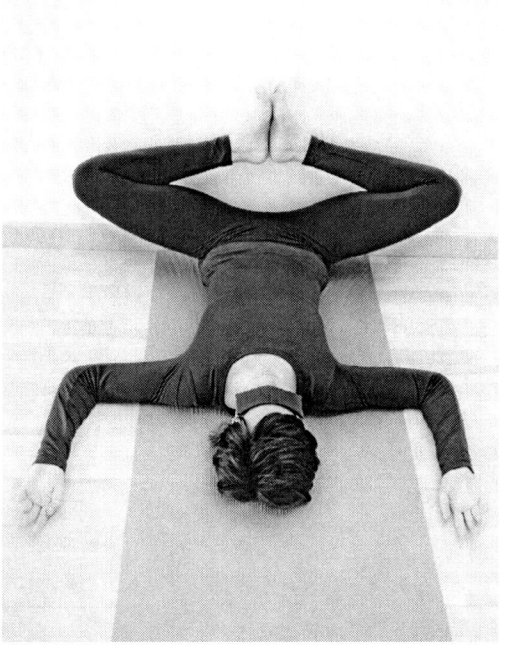
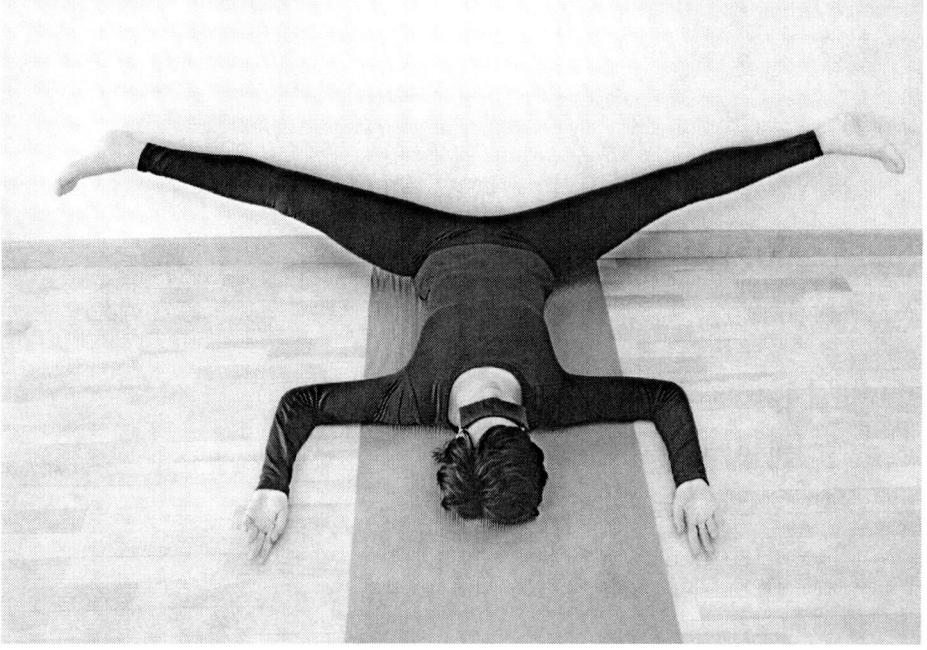

Therapeutic Applications
Depression
Exhaustion
Stress
Blood pressure

Breath in Pose
Breathe evenly and normally.

Verbal Cues
I like to use a visualization of a waterfall coming down from above and pooling in the belly, washing all the internal organs and then flowing over the chest, out the head and hands to a river that flows to the sea. These can be healing waters, crystal-filled waters, colored waters--use your imagination.
Spread the low back onto the floor and soften the back muscles.

Relieves tired or cramped legs and feet

Gently elongates the back legs, front torso and the back of the neck

Relieves mild backache

Calms the mind

Helps treat ear and eye problems

Relieves throat ailments

Helps treat kidney disorders

Contraindications

During menstruation can practice with pelvis flat on floor

Serious eye problems like glaucoma (do not practice elevated version)

Serious neck or back problems can be practiced with back directly on the floor

What to Look for With Alignment

Try to get the pelvis parallel to the floor and the legs against the wall.
Look for alignment with the body as it comes out from the wall.

Hands-on Assists

Press legs into the wall (with legs straight up the wall or in Upavista Konasana "v" legs), by straddling the torso and using your legs to gently press the legs of the practitioner into the wall.

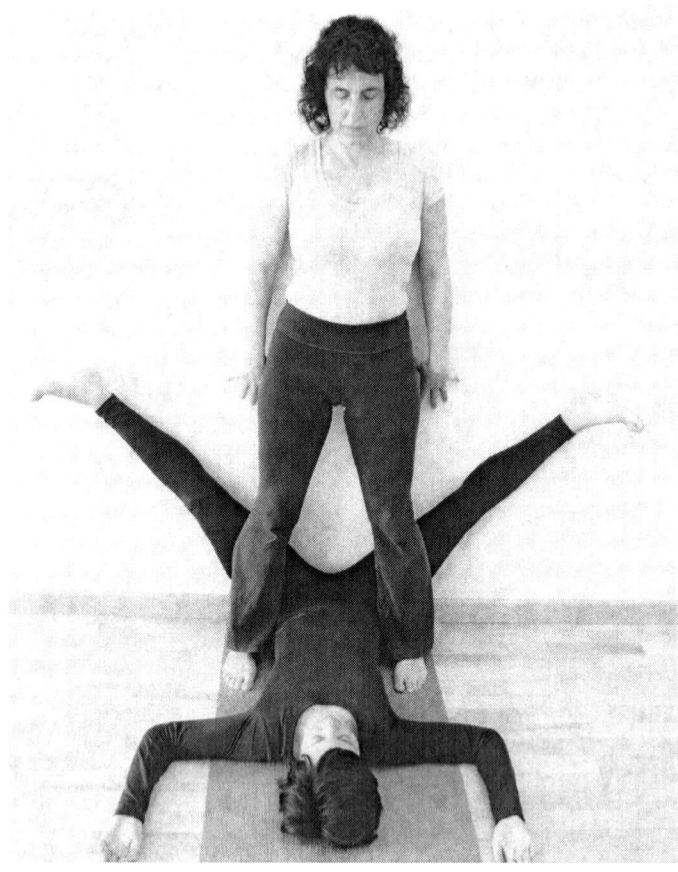

Pregnancy

This pose can be practiced in the first trimester.

How Long to Hold the Pose

3 to 20 minutes including variations

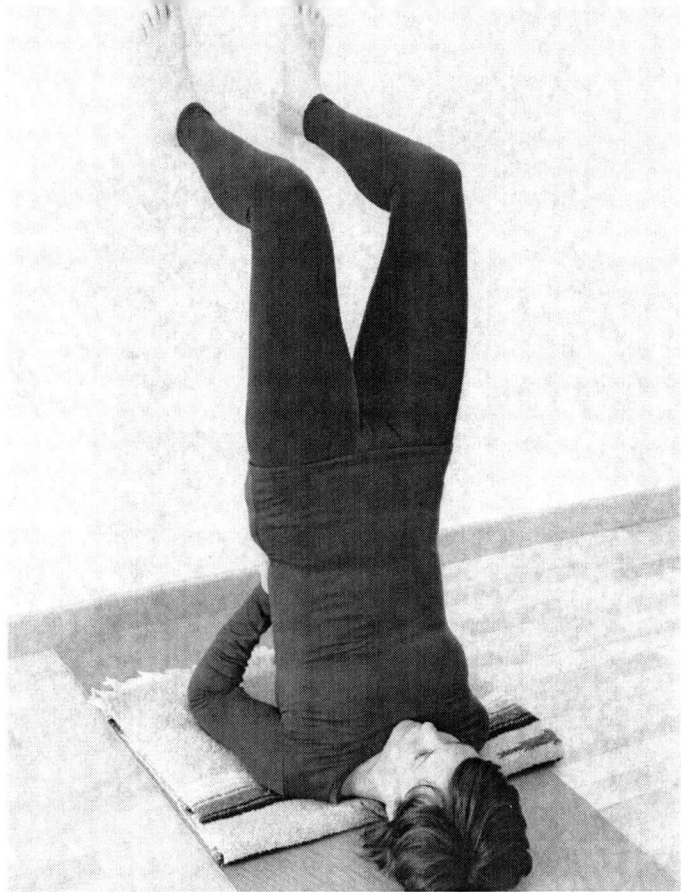

Salamba Sarvangasana (Supported Shoulder Stand)

Translation
Salamba means "propped up" and sarvanga means "all the limbs"--so we have all the limbs propped up.

General Overview
This classic asana is referred to as the "Queen of the asanas," while Sirsasana (Head Stand) is referred to as the king. It cultivates feminine energy and has so many wonderful benefits.

Basic Props Needed
Three variations:
- A wall and a mat (blanket for neck if legs come off wall)
- A chair, two mats and a bolster
- A block or bolster

Benefits

Calms the brain

Relieves stress

Relieves mild depression

Stimulates the thyroid and prostate gland

Stimulates the abdominal organs

Lengthens the shoulders and neck

Tones the legs and buttocks

Improves digestion

Helps relieve the symptoms of menopause

Reduces fatigue

Getting In and Out, On the wall

The challenge of this pose can be getting into the pose. You want to get your buttocks as close to the wall as possible. Lie down on your side with your buttocks touching the wall. This can be quite challenging for some students. Then swing the legs up the wall. Press the pelvis toward the center of the room. Keep the feet at the level of the knees. Place the feet pelvis-width apart on the wall and lift the pelvis toward the center of the room. Keep one foot on the wall and lift the other one for four breaths, then repeat on the other side. The asana may be taken into full Sarvangasana and plow Halasana if desired with or without support depending on the student. Blanket should be used under shoulders for neck support if full posture is taken. The shoulders rest on the blanket and the head on the floor. After you lift from the wall interlace the fingers under the body and bring the elbows in towards each other, then release the fingers and place the hands on the low back. Support may also be used for the feet in Halasana if the student is unable to reach the floor with the toes. Notice in the photo above how the feet are not parallel. This causes the knees to splay out slightly. I would ask this student to bring her heels out a bit to improve the alignment of the pose. One foot at a time can be lifted off the wall. This is a good variation to practice if there are neck issues. One foot always remains on the wall to keep excessive weight from resting on the neck and shoulder area.

To come out, release the hands slowly lower down, rest for a few breaths, then roll to the side and come up.

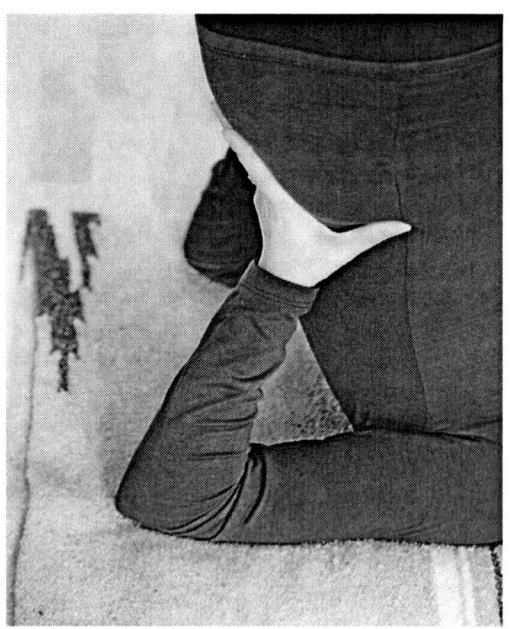

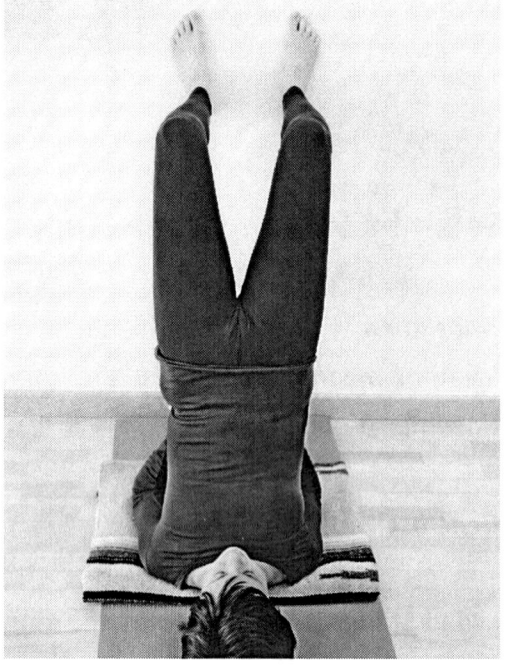

Getting In and Out, On a block(s)

Lying on the back place the feet on the floor, lift the pelvis, slide block(s) under sacrum, rest the sacrum down onto the block(s). Use one of the three heights the block offers depending on the flexibility of the practitioner. Lift the legs into the air one at a time, perpendicular to the floor.

To come out, lower the legs to the floor, press the feet into the floor, lift the pelvis and remove the block(s) from under the pelvis. Slowly release to the floor, bring the knees into the chest.

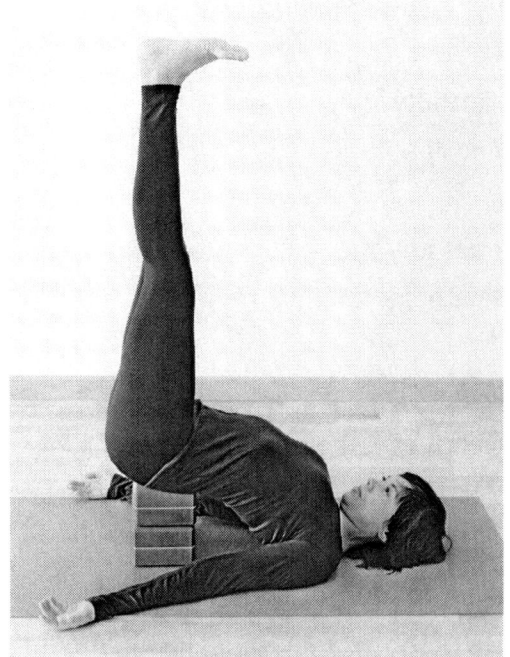

Getting In and Out, On a chair

Place a bolster below the seat of the chair and a folded mat on the chair. Sit straddling facing the back of the chair. Slide the legs up on to the back of the chair. Slide off to the edge of the chair with the feet resting on the top of the back of the chair. Hold the chair at its sides and begin to slowly lower down. Rest the shoulders on the bolster and the head on the floor. Finally lift the legs up. Hold onto the back legs on the chair.

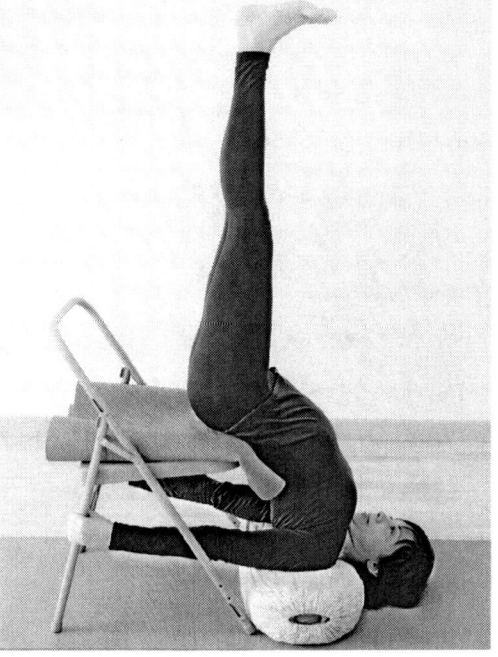

To come out, slide down onto the floor gently. Remove the bolster and place the legs on the seat of the chair. Rest for a few breaths.

Variations

Using the wall
On a block
On a chair

Alleviates insomnia

Alleviates hypertension

Soothes the nervous system

Improves bowel movements and relieves colitis

Alleviates urinary problems

Helps treat prolapsed uterus

Beneficial for varicose veins

Alleviates asthma and bronchitis

Relieves throat ailments

Supports circulatory system

Contraindications

Diarrhea

Headache

High blood pressure

Menstruation

Neck injury

Therapeutic Applications

Asthma

Infertility

Sinusitis

Breath in Pose

Breathe normally through the nose.

Verbal Cues

Feel the energy running down the legs. Sense the thyroid gland being washed with blood and fresh energy.

What to Look for With Alignment

Check the neck and head for alignment. Check that the elbows are in alignment with the shoulders.

Hands-on Assists

Bring the elbows in.

For pregnancy, swollen ankle and leg massage.

Pregnancy

If you are experienced with this pose, you can continue to practice it late into pregnancy. I suggest using the legs on the wall version for pregnant woman in the second and third trimesters. The legs can be elevated one leg at a time for 2-4 breaths on each side. (See p. 140 for more information about this posture during pregnancy.)

How Long to Hold the Pose

30 seconds to 10 minutes

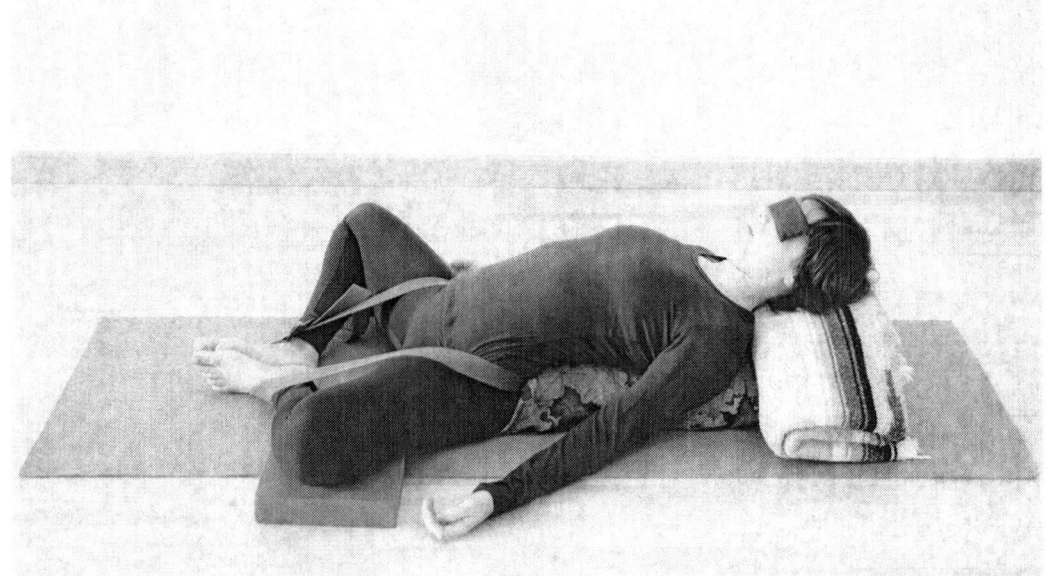

Supine (Lying Down) and Twists

Supta Baddha Konasana (Reclining Bound Angle Pose)

Translation

Supta means "reclining," baddha means "fixed" or "bound" and kona means "angle."

General Overview

This is one of the most popular restorative postures. Enjoyed by almost all students with variations to accommodate individual concerns. Next to Savasana it is the most widely practiced restorative posture.

Basic Props Needed

Bolster, two blocks (or two blankets or two cushions), one folded blanket (or small pillow), belt, eye bag and blanket to cover the body. This can also be done with four blocks, one for head, one for shoulders and two for thigh support.

Getting In

Sit in Baddha Konasana, soles of the feet joined and knees splaying out to the sides with the short end of your bolster behind you and your two blocks (or folded blankets or cushions) under your knees enough to support the inner groin; there should be no pulling felt on the inner thighs. Place a blanket on the end of your bolster to rest your head on. Make a loop in your belt and place the belt around your body on the low back sacral

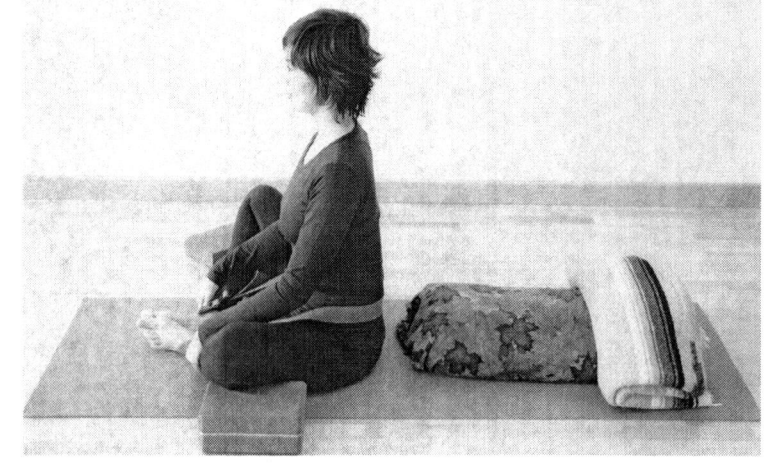

97

Benefits

Regulates blood pressure

Soothes and tones the digestive system

Tones the kidneys

Improves blood circulation in the ovary area

Helps to balance the reproductive organs during puberty, menstruation and menopause

Relieves menstrual pain

Relieves varicose veins

Relieves sciatica

Helps corrects a prolapsed uterus

Reduces the pain caused by hemorrhoids

Softens hips and groins

Helps to alleviate depression

Helps to relieve anxiety

Opens the chest and heart

Opens the front of the body

area, then down over the inside of your knees, and then around and under your feet. Using your hands and arms to help you, slowly lie back onto the bolster. Adjust the blanket to rest under your head. Place your eye bag over your eyes.

Getting Out

To come out of the pose, place your hands palms down on the floor, and in one movement using your hands to support you lift your head in the direction of your chest and sit up.

Variations for Different Concerns

Low Back Discomfort: There are several adjustments to make to relieve low back discomfort. Move the bolster a few inches away from the lower back sacral area then lie back. Move the feet out several inches away from the body.

Use a smaller bolster or lower the height of the support the student will lie back on by using a single folded blanket.

Adjust the bolster by placing something under the end farthest away from the head, creating an upward angle up to 45 degrees. This variation should also be used with pregnant woman in their second and third trimesters.

Adjust the neck (head level).

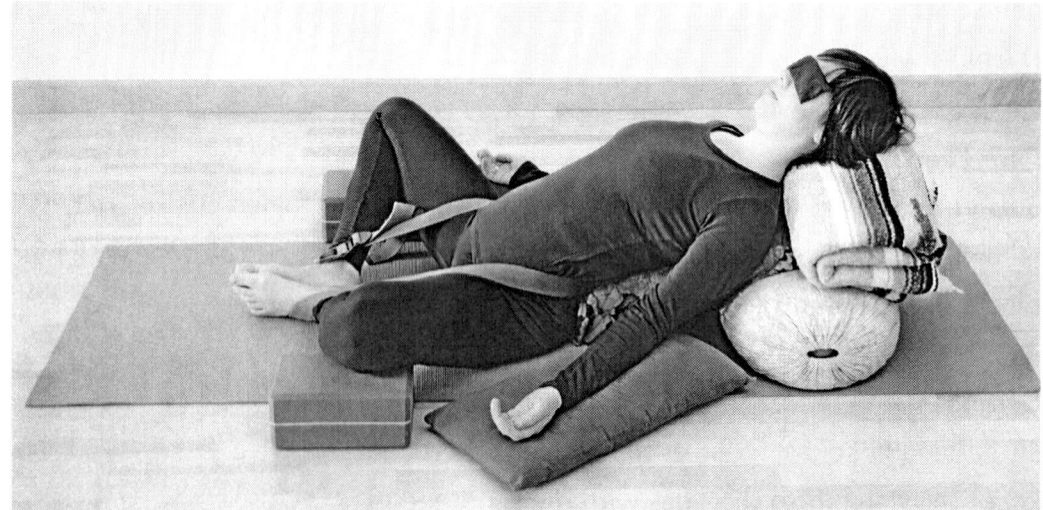

Shoulder Discomfort: Place folded blankets or small pillows under the arms.

Neck Discomfort: Make sure the head is fully supported and check the angle of the head and neck for alignment. Work with adjusting the head level until the student is comfortable. The throat should be soft and relaxed.

Inner Thigh or Groin Discomfort: Make sure the inner thighs are fully supported by placing more support under the bent legs. If this doesn't remedy the situation extend the legs out and rest them flat on the floor or over a bolster or blanket. *Knee Discomfort:* Depending on the level of discomfort and mobility: First try using more support under the knees; if this does not alleviate the discomfort allow the legs to rest forward flat on the floor or with a bolster under the bottom of the lower thigh/upper knee area.

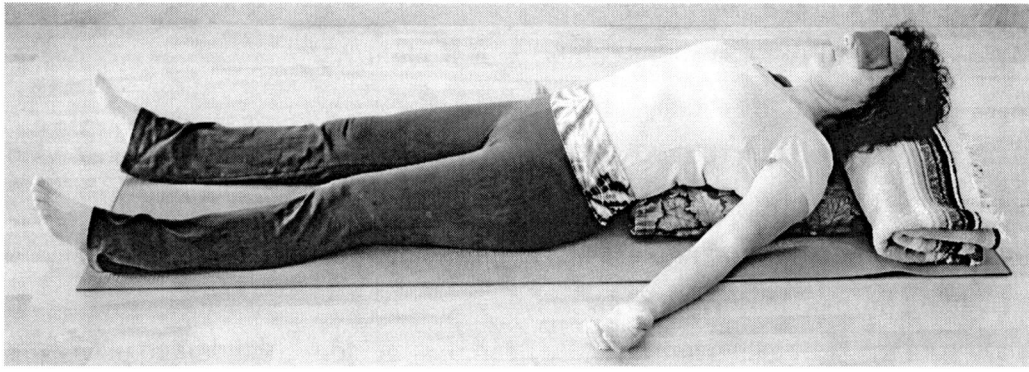

Contraindications

If you have spondylolisthesis, spondylolysis or diagnosed disc disease

If there is pain in the back that cannot be remedied by variations

After 3 months of pregnancy must practice with variation

Therapeutic Applications
Stress
PMS
Menstruation
Menopause
Depression
Anxiety
Digestion
Blood pressure

Breath in Pose
I will often guide students to breathe into their chests and expand the upper body while this area is being accentuated by the bolster. When not focusing on any particular way of breathing the breath is soft and natural through the nose. Other pranayama techniques can be practiced while resting in the pose including Valoma 2 Pranayama: exhale gently, then hold the breath out for 2 seconds before inhaling; do this 3 to 5 times. Never strain when doing pranayama; if you feel out of breath or strained in any way resume breathing normally. After your breath has normalized you can return to complete your pranayama.

Verbal Cues
Bring your shoulder blades together and down your back.

Take your hands to the flesh of your buttocks and slide the flesh towards your feet, opening a space in your low back.

Visualize a bud of a flower in your heart chakra and see it opening up into full bloom in slow motion, one petal at a time, or slowly opening all the petals at once.

What to Look for With Alignment

Make sure the bolster is straight behind your student.

Make sure their feet are even, big toe to heel.

Make sure the strap is in the correct place on the sacral part of the back and looped or connected correctly.

There should be an even angular line from forehead to nose, to chest to belly, to feet, going from up to down evenly.

Make sure the body is in a line laterally, head to shoulders, shoulders to pelvis and pelvis to feet.

Hands-on Assists

Moving the shoulder blades, in and down: Flattening and releasing the shoulders and shoulder blades. This is done inviting the student to relax completely then sliding the hands under the shoulder blades and directing them in and down. A massage may be given to the rhomboids (the muscles located between the shoulder blades and spine) when hands are under the shoulders.

Thumbs in three points in shoulders: Press the thumbs into the tops of the shoul-

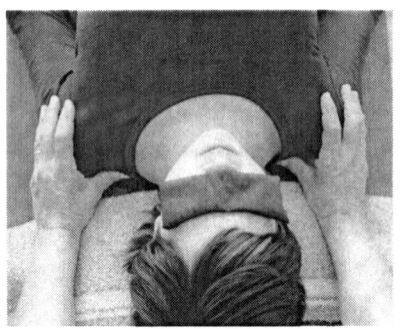

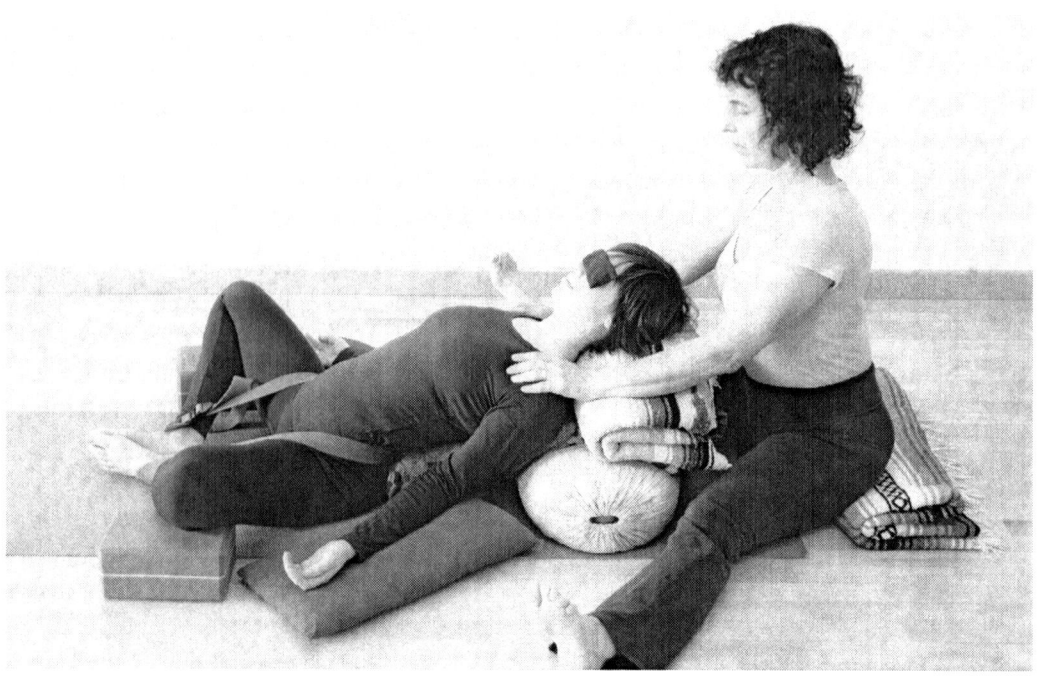

ders starting close to the neck and moving out towards the arms. Press on the fleshy area, not on the bone.

Gentle neck pull: Hold the head with hands, fingertips under the occipital ridge, and pull the head towards you gently.

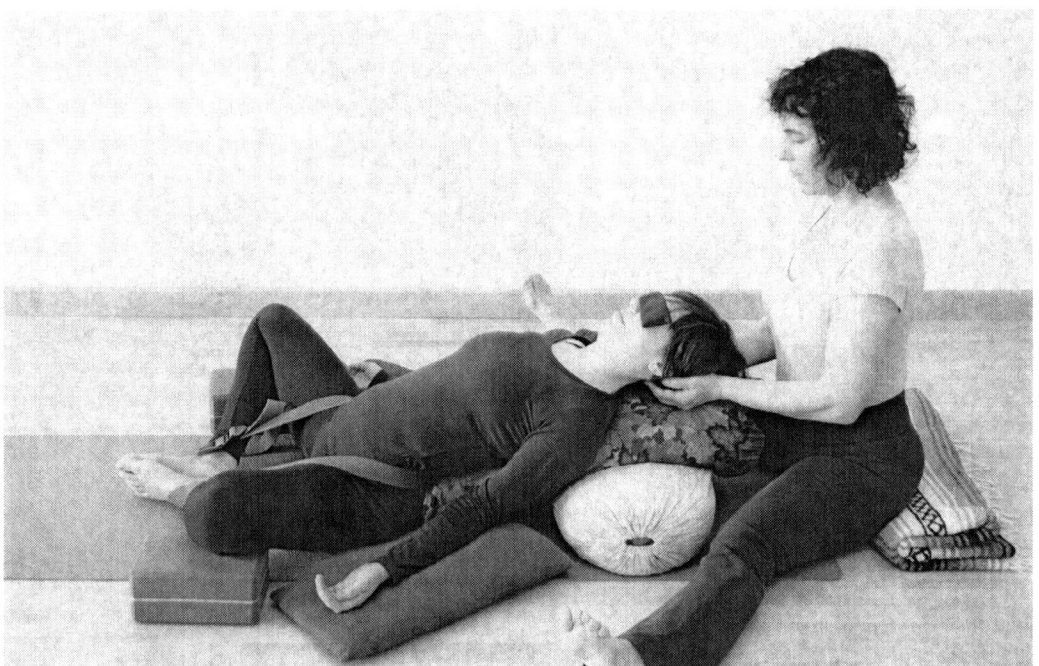
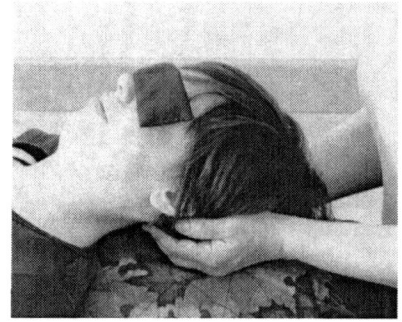

Head hold: Hold the head gently in your hands and encourage deep relaxation of the head into the hands. For occipital ridge release, place the fingers on the neck just below the occipital ridge and allow the student's head to relax in your hands and their neck to soften into your fingers.

Hand massage: Giving a simple hand massage while your student is resting can be a powerful way to encourage deeper relaxation.

Arm swing: Taking your student's wrist and lifting their arm, gently swing the arm back and forth. If they are not fully relaxed you will feel them holding the arm. Encourage them to let go and to make their arm heavy. If they are unable to relax their arm, take the elbow and wrist, supporting their arm more fully with small gentle movements and continue to encourage them to let go. Then gently release their arm back to the earth. Often they will be able to surrender and relax, but if they are not able simply encourage them to continue to be aware and to practice relaxation.

Foot massage: (when legs are extended) This can be as simple as holding the feet for a few moments.

Aura circle around heart: Sitting behind your student with your hands about 5 or 6 inches above the heart and with the palms facing towards your student's body, make a circle in the air creating the shape of a circle above and around their hearts.

Allow each hand to make a circle in an inward direction--the right hand will circle from right to left and the left hand will circle from left to right. The circles will overlap each other over the student's heart.

Heart to neck or head polarity: Gently and softly place one hand behind the student's neck and the other on their heart center. Energy flows out through the right hand and in through the left. You can imagine the energy circulating from and to your hands and through your student's heart in a circuit of healing or light or love. Become a conduit of energy.

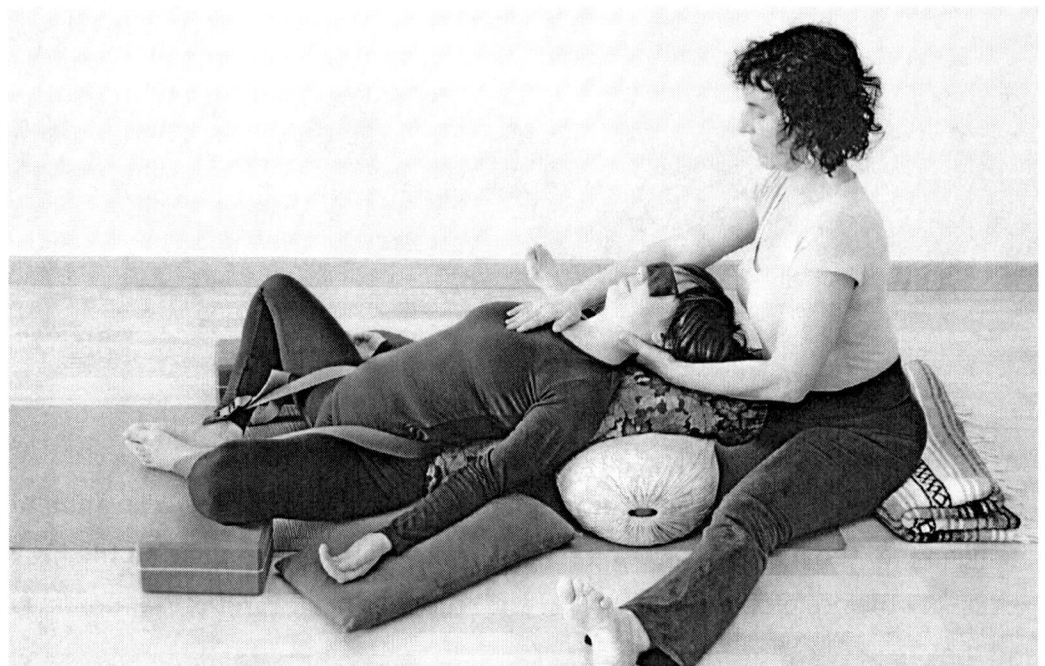

Pregnancy

In second and third trimesters this pose can be modified to create an angle that keeps the womb from pressing on the vena cava which runs along the inside of the spine on the right side. Extra support is needed under the back and the arms. (See p. 143 for more information about this posture during pregnancy.)

How Long to Hold the Pose
2 to 25 minutes

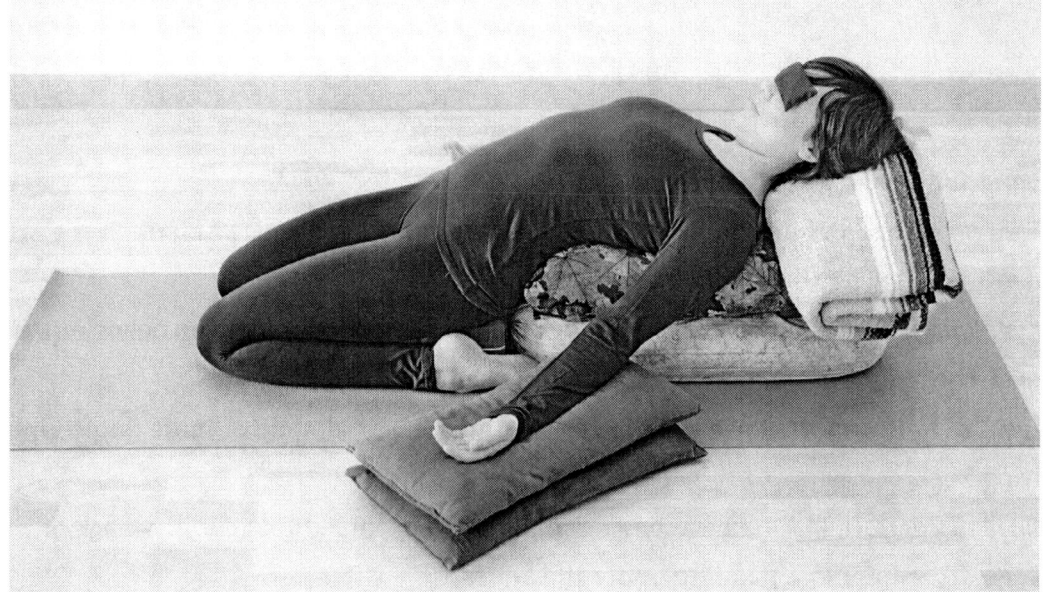

Supta Virasana (Reclining Hero Pose)

Translation
Supta means "lying down" and Vira means "hero" or "champion."

General Overview
This is a beneficial posture that can be challenging for some students. With patience and understanding of how to use the support of props it can be practiced by many and the benefits are plentiful.

Basic Props Needed
Bolster(s), blanket and often block(s)and eye bag(s)

Getting In
Determine how much support is needed to sit with comfort in Virasana. With that amount of support under the pelvis and possibly a bit more depending on the openness of the quadriceps, build up the support behind the student with bolsters and other props so that they can lie back supported without discomfort. If you have created a bit of an angle place something under the forearms as shown in the photo above to create support for the shoulders. Slowly lie back using the arms for support.

Getting Out
To come out use the arms to help, pressing the hands into the floor as you bring the chin towards the chest and sit up in one smooth movement.

Variations for Different Concerns

This pose may require many props to create comfort for your student. Some students will not be able to practice this asana.

Knee and ankle discomfort: Place a block or two as needed under the pelvis, equally raise the height of the bolsters to support the back fully.

Low back discomfort: Raise the bolster(s) to create a 45-degree or more angle when lying back.

Knee discomfort: Place an eye bag or small rolled or folded towel in the back of the knee. Try using more padding under the knees.

Therapeutic Applications

Arthritis

Asthma

Digestive problems

Flat feet

Headache

High blood pressure

Infertility

Insomnia

Menstrual problems

Respiratory ailments

Sciatica

Varicose veins

Knee problems

Breath in Pose

Breathe into the front of the body.

Breathe into the rib cage and chest.

Breathe normally.

Verbal Cues

Feel the front of the body opening.

What to Look for With Alignment

Check for the bolster being aligned under the body.

Check for the angle of support from the lower to the upper ends of the body.

Benefits

Opens the abdomen

Elongates the thighs and deep hip flexors (psoas), knees, and ankles

Strengthens the arches

Helps correct flat feet

Relieves tired legs

Improves digestion

Helps relieve the symptoms of menstrual pain

Helps prevent arterial blockages

Check for the foot position on both sides, toenails touching the floor, heels facing upwards towards the sky.

Check for feet resting at the sides of the thighs, not under.

Check that the thighs are parallel and connected to each other.

Hands-on Assists

Head hold and Gentle neck pull (see pp. 38, 39 for more details).

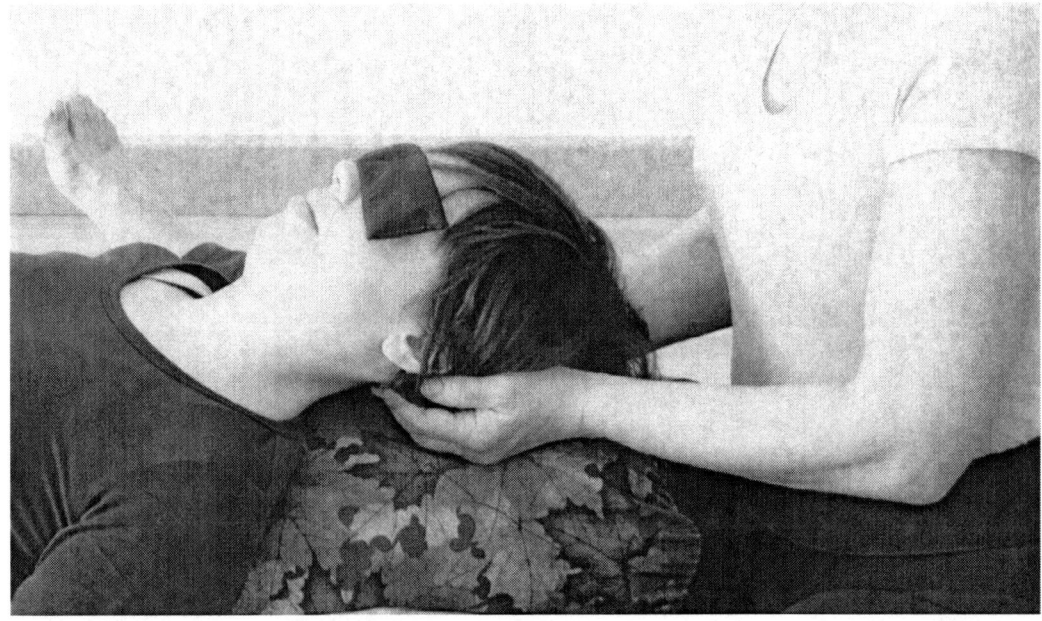

Thumbs in three points in shoulders: Press the thumbs into the three points in the

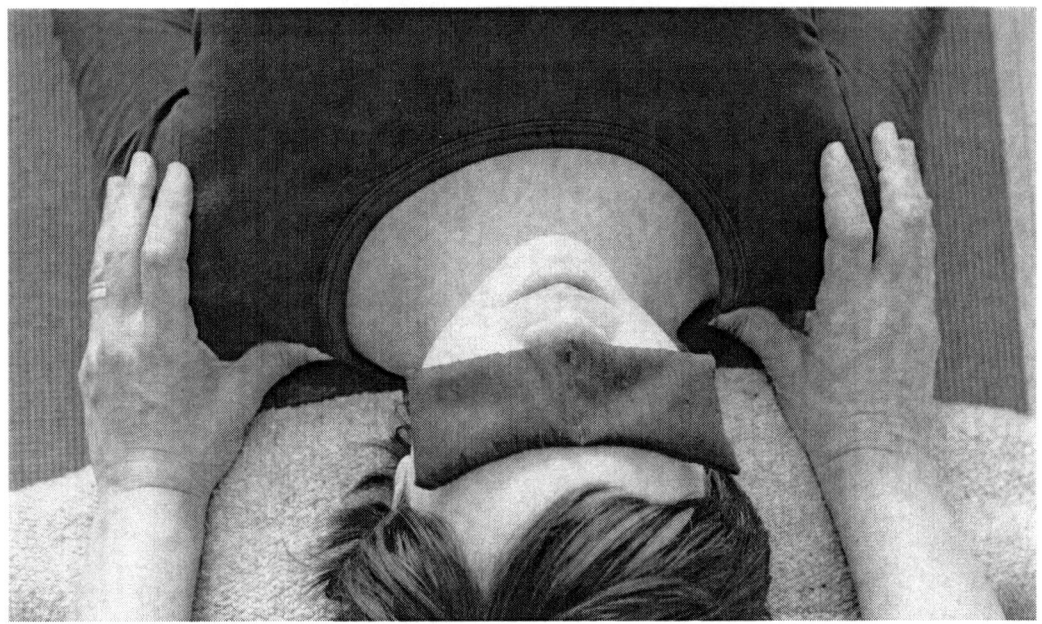

tops of the shoulders (see page 39).

Increases the elasticity of lung tissue

Enhances resistance to infections

Relieves indigestion, acidity and flatulence

Corrects a prolapsed uterus, and tones the pelvic organs

Reduces inflammation in the knees, and relieves gout and rheumatic pain

Relieves pain and fatigue in the legs

Feet, kidney point press: Press your fist or thumb into the bottom center of the foot just below the ball of the foot.

Pregnancy

In the second and third trimesters the pose can be modified to create an angle of a minimum of 30 to 45 degrees that keeps the womb from pressing on the vena cava (the major vein that brings blood to the baby) which runs along the inside of the spine on the right side. (See p. 148 for more information about this posture during pregnancy.)

How Long to Hold the Pose
30 seconds to 10 minutes

Contraindications

If there are any serious back, knee or ankle problems, or pain in the knees, ankles, feet or low back that cannot be remedied by variations to support these areas avoid this pose

Do not practice if there are problems with a serious heart condition, partially blocked arteries, angina or if the student is recovering from bypass surgery

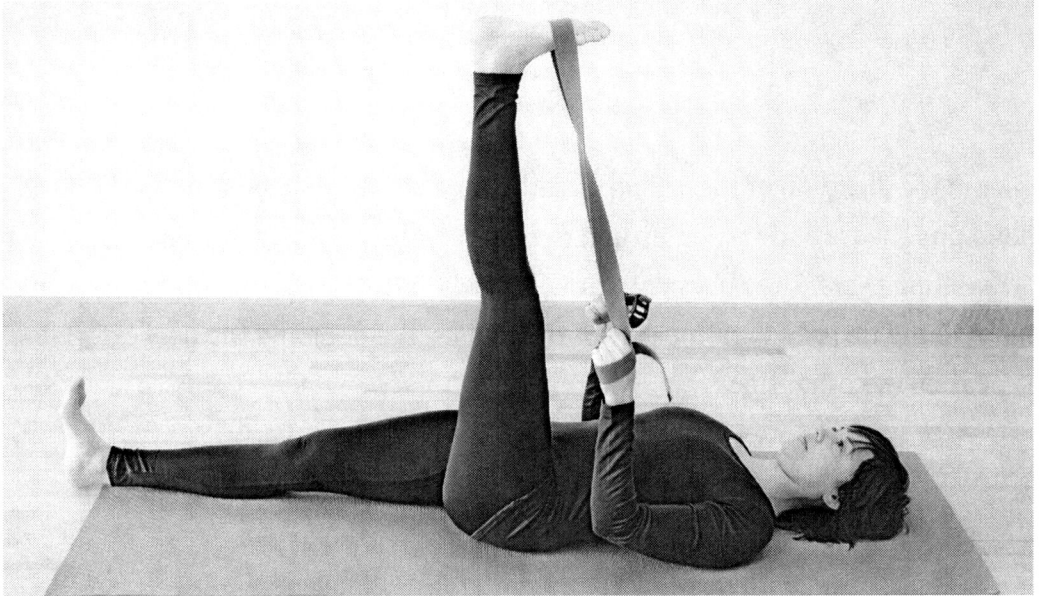

Supported Supta Padangusthasana (Reclining Big Toe Pose)

Translation

Supta means "lying down" or "lying back," pada means "foot" and angustha means "big toe," and so the pose is called Reclining Big Toe Pose.

General Overview

This is a great pose for those who have tight hips and or hamstrings. With its variations to both sides it can affect the legs, hips, pelvis and back in a very positive manner.

Basic Props Needed

Yoga strap, bolster and/or blocks for both sides

Getting In and Out

This pose has three parts per side. Lie with the back on a mat on the floor, legs extended through the heels. If the head doesn't rest comfortably on the floor, support it on a folded blanket or small pillow. Pull the right heel towards the chest and place the tie around the ball of the foot; straighten the foot to the sky. Breathe for 2 to 5 or more breaths. Make sure the tie is wrapped around the hands and the collarbones are wide and open. (See photo above for arm and tie position.)

Take both ends of the tie in the right hand, open the leg out to the right so the full side of the foot is supported by a prop(s). Externally rotate the right thigh and extend through both heels. The left arm rests out to the left side and head and eyes gaze in the direction of the ceiling. Breathe for 2 to 5 or more breaths. With the left hand pull the tie and the leg up and over to the other side, resting on prop(s) that are waiting there. The pelvis will come off the floor on one side and the foot that is not in the tie rests with the side of the foot on the floor and the heel extending. Repeat on the other side.

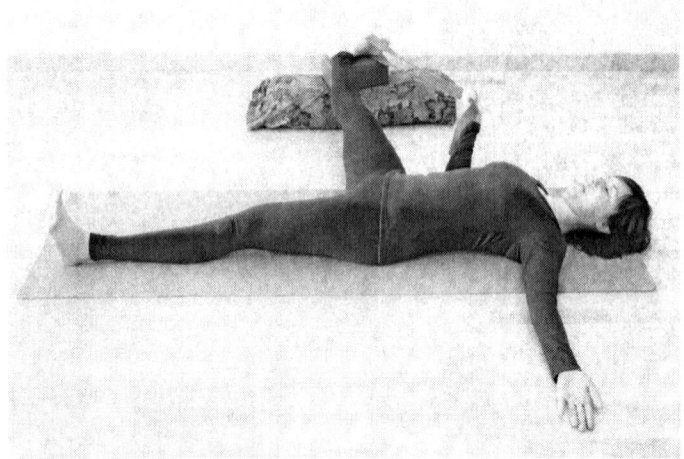
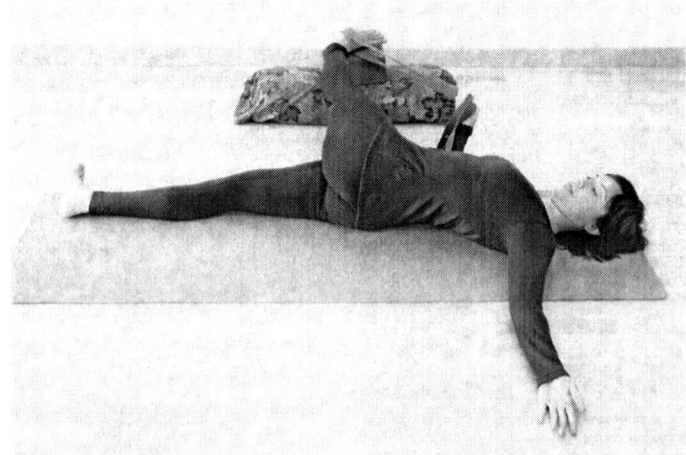

Variations for Different Concerns
Inner thigh discomfort: Support the foot resting out to the side more.
Practice with the foot on the floor against a wall.
Place a blanket under the head if needed.
If the head rests easily on the floor with no neck discomfort do not support the head.

Benefits

Opens the knees

Improves digestion

Relieves backache

Relieves sciatica

Relieves menstrual discomfort

Open hips, thighs, hamstrings, groins and calves

Therapeutic Applications
Osteoarthritis of the hips and knees
Sciatica
Menstrual pain
Back pain

Breath in Pose
Breathe into any sensation, tension or holding and soften

Verbal Cues
Draw your thighbone in towards the pelvis (when the leg is extended upward).
Press out through both heels.
Firm the muscles in the legs, press out through the heels, then relax gently with the support at the sides.

What to Look for With Alignment

Look for evenness to the midline.

See that the arms are supported in the twisting variation and not hanging in the air. If there isn't enough flexibility for the arm to rest back to the floor have the student rest the arm on the side of their body.

Hands-on Assists

First part: Ground the leg that is resting on the floor with a foot. Stand with the student's up-stretched leg in front of you. Adjust the tie onto the ball of the foot to help them to straighten their knee and depending on their flexibility encourage the leg to open. Help them to have the bottom of the foot facing the ceiling if possible.

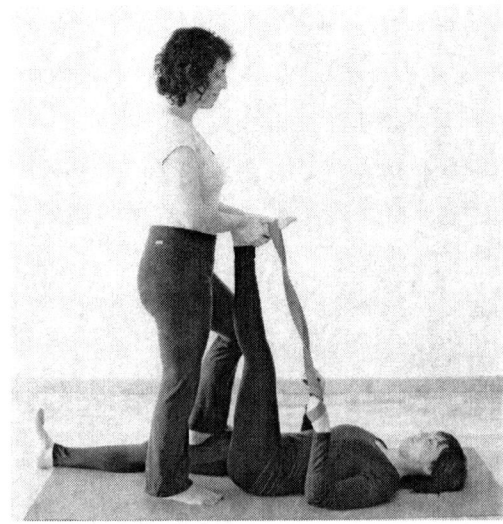

Second part: Help to externally rotate the leg extended to the side with a gentle hand on the thigh above the knee and encourage an outward rotation of the thigh if needed.

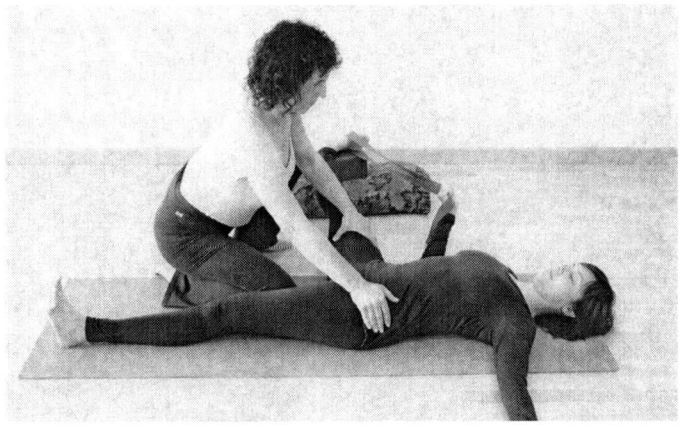

Third part: Assist with the twist by placing one hand on the hip and the other on the upper arm or shoulder and gently encourage the natural curve in the lower back.

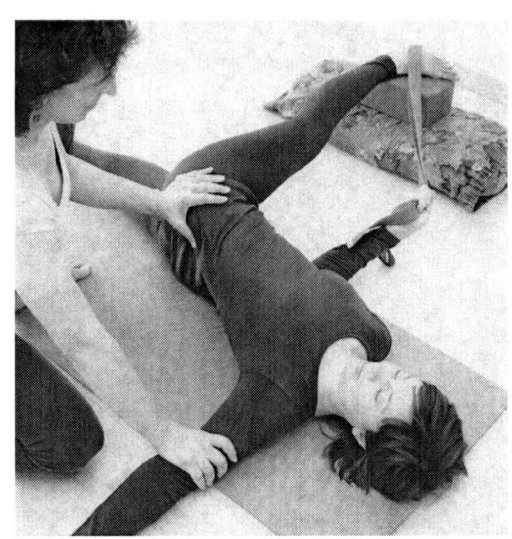

Contraindications

Diarrhea

Headache

High blood pressure: Raise the head and neck on a folded blanket.

Recovering from heart condition or blocked arteries

Pregnancy
Only practice in the first trimester the first and second variations, if a regular yoga practice is established. Do not practice in the second and third trimesters.

How Long to Hold the Pose
20 seconds to 3 minutes on each side

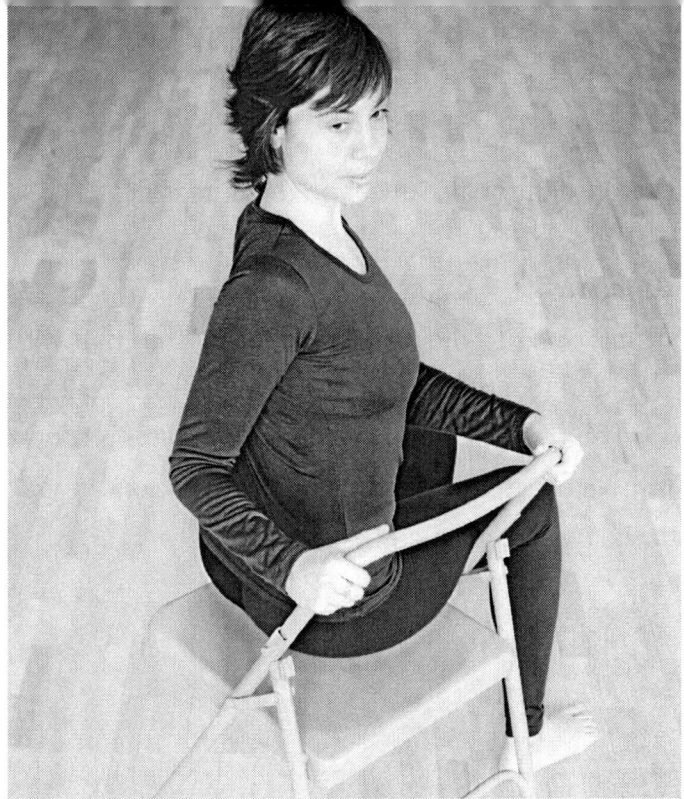

Utthita Marichyasana (Seated and Standing Twist with Chair)

Translation
Marichi means a "ray of light" and was a great sage, the son of Brahma, the creator of the universe.

General Overview
These poses can help to relieve backache, shoulder and neck pain and keep the spine supple.

Basic Props Needed
Chair, wall

Getting In and Out, Sitting variation
Sit on the chair so that the back of the chair is at your right side.
Place the feet parallel to each other on the floor. If the floor is too far for the feet to rest flat on the floor place blocks under the feet. If the floor is too close place blankets on the chair so that the thighs rest parallel to the floor and hip-width apart. With your upper body turn to the right so that you can hold the sides of the back of the chair. Use the hands to help you to enter into the twist by pulling on the left

hand and pushing the right hand into the chair. Repeat on the other side.

Benefits

Supports digestion

Relieves low back pain

Opens the shoulders and neck

Keeps the spine supple

Getting In and Out, Standing variation

Place the chair (small stool or table) next to the wall. Stand facing the chair with the wall on your right. Place your right foot on the chair, turn towards the wall and place your fingertips on the wall at chest height; keeping your upper body over your pelvis turn to the right from sacrum to the head, using the hands on the wall to assist you in deepening into the twist. Repeat on the left side.

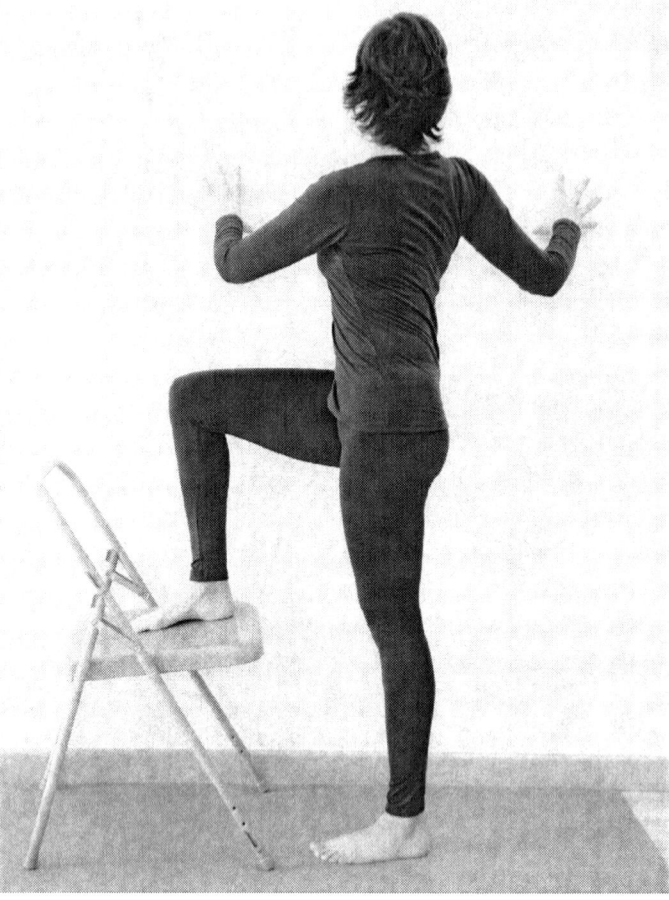

Variations for Different Concerns

Most students can practice these positions without any variation.

Therapeutic Applications

Shoulder and neck pain

Breath in Pose

Breathe through the whole torso and down into the pelvis. Full, deep breath in twisting poses massages the organs and the lymphatic system. Take 2-5 deep breaths, then breathe normally.

Verbal Cues
Standing variation: Press the hands gently into the wall as you lift your chest and draw your shoulders blades in and down the back.
On the chair: Use the hands to press and pull to increase the twist.

What to Look for With Alignment
Make sure the thighs and feet are parallel to each other and a hip-width apart. A block can be placed between the knees to help with stabilizing the legs and keep them aligned.

Hands-on Assists
Place the flats of your hands on the shoulders and upper back and gently encourage the shoulder blades to move in and down the back.

Pregnancy
Not to be practiced after the first trimester. Practice in the first trimester if a regular yoga practice is established.

How Long to Hold the Pose
15 seconds to 1 minute on each side.

Contraindications

High or low blood pressure

Serious cardiac condition

Migraine

A cold or bronchitis

Diarrhea or constipation

Osteoarthritis of the knees for standing variation; seated variation is fine

Heavy menstruation

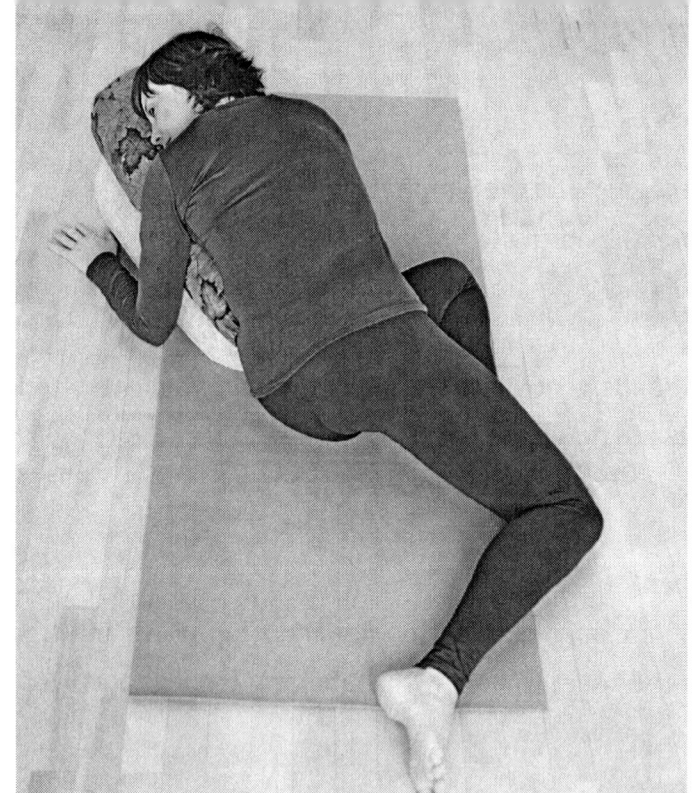

Balasana with Twist
(Face Down Forward Reclining Twist with a Bolster)

Translation
Balasana is the "pose of the child." This variation is done with a twist through the pelvis and torso.

General Overview
A great pose to release stress in the back, neck and shoulder muscles, massage organs and lymphs with the breath and stretch the intercostal muscles of the rib cage.

Basic Props Needed
Two bolsters, or two blocks under one bolster, and a wall for the wall variation

Getting In and Out
Sit with the knees to the right side and right foot resting on the left thigh. Place the short end of the bolster resting on the right hip extending out from the pelvis the long way. Turn to the right and place the hands on either side of the bolster, extend the torso then lie down with the belly and front of the body having as

Benefits

Lengthens the spine

Opens the shoulders and hips

Massages the abdominal organs

Relieves sciatica

Helps relieve stress

Improves digestion

Relieves lower backache and neck pain

much contact with the bolster as possible, and the forearms on the floor turning the head to the left for less twist and the right for more of a twist. Switch sides. On the wall create a box with the right foot on the wall and the left shin resting on the wall with the left toes pointed. Lie over the bolster in the same way as above. Switch sides.

In both variations try to get the front of the body from the pubic bone to the top of the head resting on the bolster. To come out place the hands under the shoulders and push up.

Variations for Different Concerns

Adjust the angle and height of the bolster to increase or decrease the angle and height of the twist.

Low Back Discomfort: Raise the bolster height and work with the angle of the bolster to the pelvis.

Neck Discomfort: keep the head turned to the side the knees are pointing or place a support, block or blanket or cushion, under the forehead.

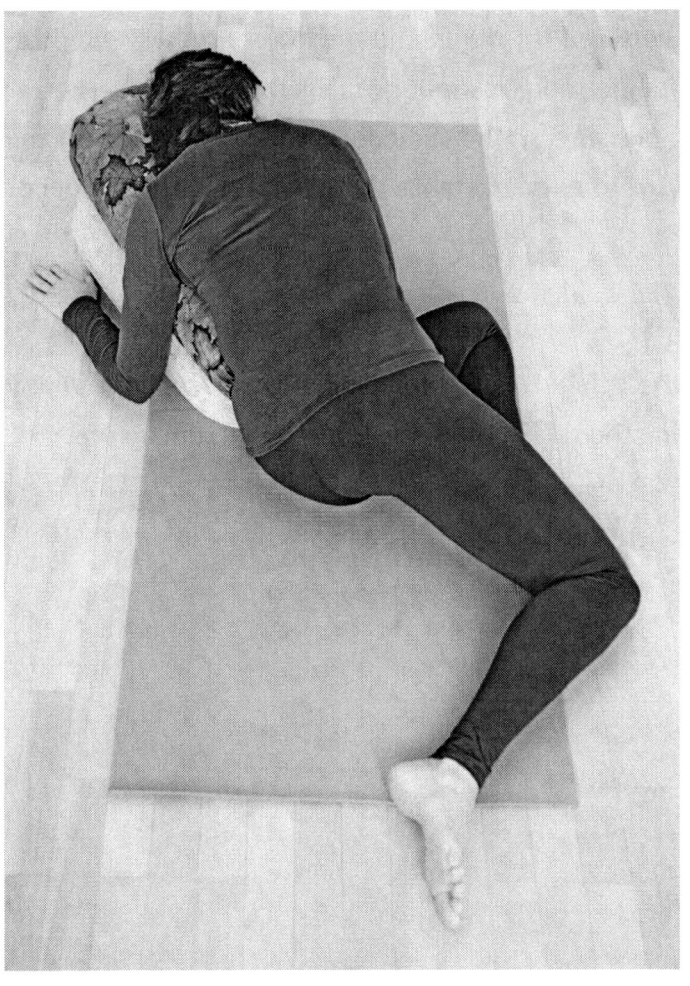

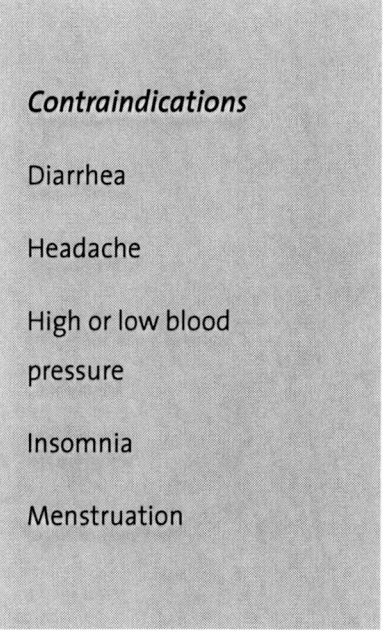

Contraindications

Diarrhea

Headache

High or low blood pressure

Insomnia

Menstruation

Therapeutic Applications

Carpel tunnel syndrome

Stress

Breath in Pose

Deep breath, followed by normal breathing

Verbal Cues

Feel the body expand with the incoming breath, know that your organs are being massaged from the inside out as you twist and breathe.

What to Look for With Alignment

When practicing against the wall look for right angles with feet and lower and upper legs. Check that the bolster is positioned correctly, supporting as much of the torso as possible from the pubic bone to top of the head.

Check that the forearms are resting on the floor and there is no crunching in the shoulder.

Check for a 45-degree angle between the upper and the lower arm with no pressure on the shoulders. If a 45-degree angle cannot be taken make sure elbows rest out to the sides without any pressure on the shoulders. If the elbows are off the ground place blankets under the forearms to make them parallel with the floor or use a smaller bolster.

Hands-on Assists

Massage on either side of the spine: Follow the spine with the fingers, gently pressing into the muscles along the side of the spine from the sacrum up the back. Encourage twist and elongation.

Pregnancy

Do not practice.

How Long to Hold the Pose

20 seconds to 2 minutes on each side

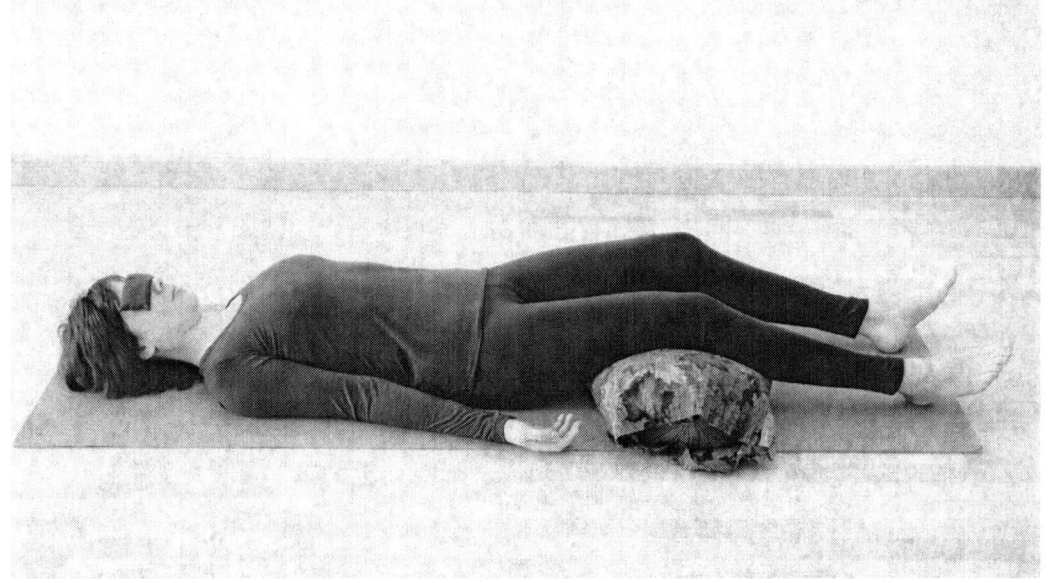

Savasana (Corpse Pose)

Translation

Sava means "corpse" and asana means "pose"; it is sometimes called Dead Man's Pose.

General Overview

This is one of the most basic and important restorative poses as it can be practiced anywhere without the need of props. Deep relaxation can be achieved and many benefits can be gained.

Basic Props Needed

Head support if needed, but only if there are neck problems.
Bolster or rolled blanket under the knees particulary if there are low back issues.
Blanket for cover if needed and eye bag.

Getting In and Out

Lie down on your back face up on a mat or blanket. The arms are at the sides of the body and the palms facing up. The feet are a comfortable distance apart, a bit wider than the pelvis, toes resting out to the sides. If using support for the legs place it below the lower thigh/upper knee area of the legs.

Contraindications

Variation for pregnancy in second and third trimesters: side lying with support (see photo p. 119)

Variations for Different Concerns
Low back discomfort: Place a bolster or folded blankets under the bottom of the thighs. Lie completely flat on the floor with no props at all.

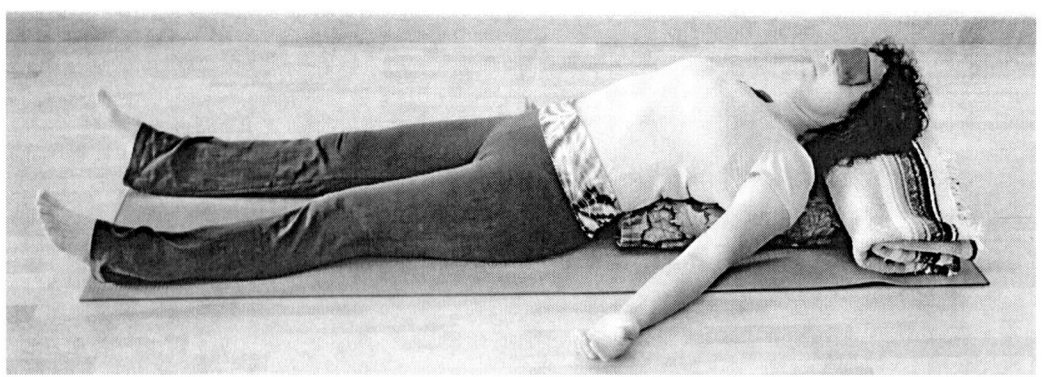

Benefits

Calms the brain

Relaxes the body

Promotes inner peace and tranquility

Supports immune system function

Soothes the nervous system

Releases stress

Reduces headache

Alleviates fatigue

Alleviates insomnia

Increases mental clarity

Improves memory

Therapeutic Applications
Stress
Depression
Recovery from illness
Anxiety

Breath in Pose
Normal gentle breath

Verbal Cues
This pose can be led with a progressive relaxation and other visualizations.
Feel the brain moving away from the front of the skull.

What to Look for With Alignment
Look for the body to be in one line, the palms face upward and the feet slightly apart with feet falling to the outside. The feet should be on the floor and not hanging in the air if the lower thighs/knees are being supported. If more support is being used under the knees for back issues, place support under the feet also so they are not hanging.
Check all parts of the body for alignment and evenness.

Hands-on Assists
Observe the head of your student and its position in relationship to the shoulders. Sometimes students' heads can be tilted or turned to one side or the other. Gently

cradle the head in your hands and draw the base of the skull away from the back of the neck, lengthening the back of the neck, so that the head rests evenly. Gently lay the head back down on the floor or support, making sure that the tip of their nose is pointing directly toward the ceiling and the head is not tilted forward or back or to either side. If the chin protrudes up place support under the head to compensate.

Shoulder press with palms and finger press of three points in shoulders.

Pull feet at the heel away from the head; rock the body while holding feet.

Massage the feet or hands.

Massage (wipe) the forehead. Place the palms in the center of the forehead and with a gentle pressure move the palms away from one another.

Release the jaw by placing the fingertips gently on the sides of the face on the bottom of the jaw. Very lightly with the tips of the fingers encourage a down and slightly forward movement.

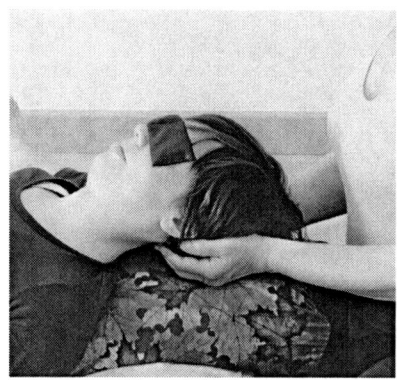

Pregnancy

Lie down on side with support under the head; support between the legs, letting the leg on top be supported so that the foot is higher than the heart; support under belly (baby) as needed and support for the upper arm. If needed back support is also recommended. (See p. 151 for more information about this posture during pregnancy.)

How Long to Hold the Pose

2 to 30 minutes

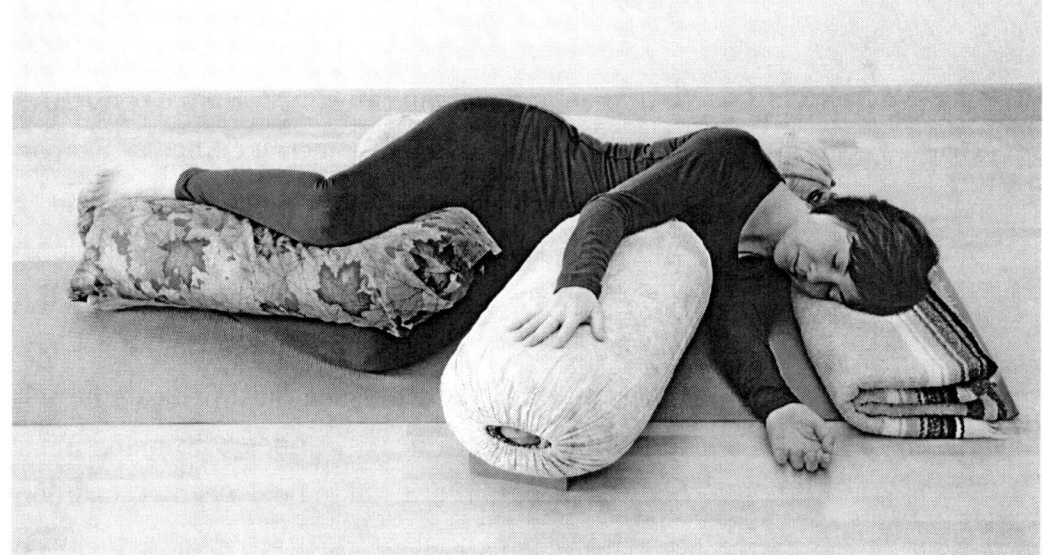

Increases concentration

Helps to regulate blood pressure

Improves circulation to and function of organs and organ systems

Alleviates discomforts associated with menstruation, pregnancy and menopause

Reduces anxiety

Reduces depression

Reduces dependency on medications

Supports the recovery from illness

CHAPTER 11

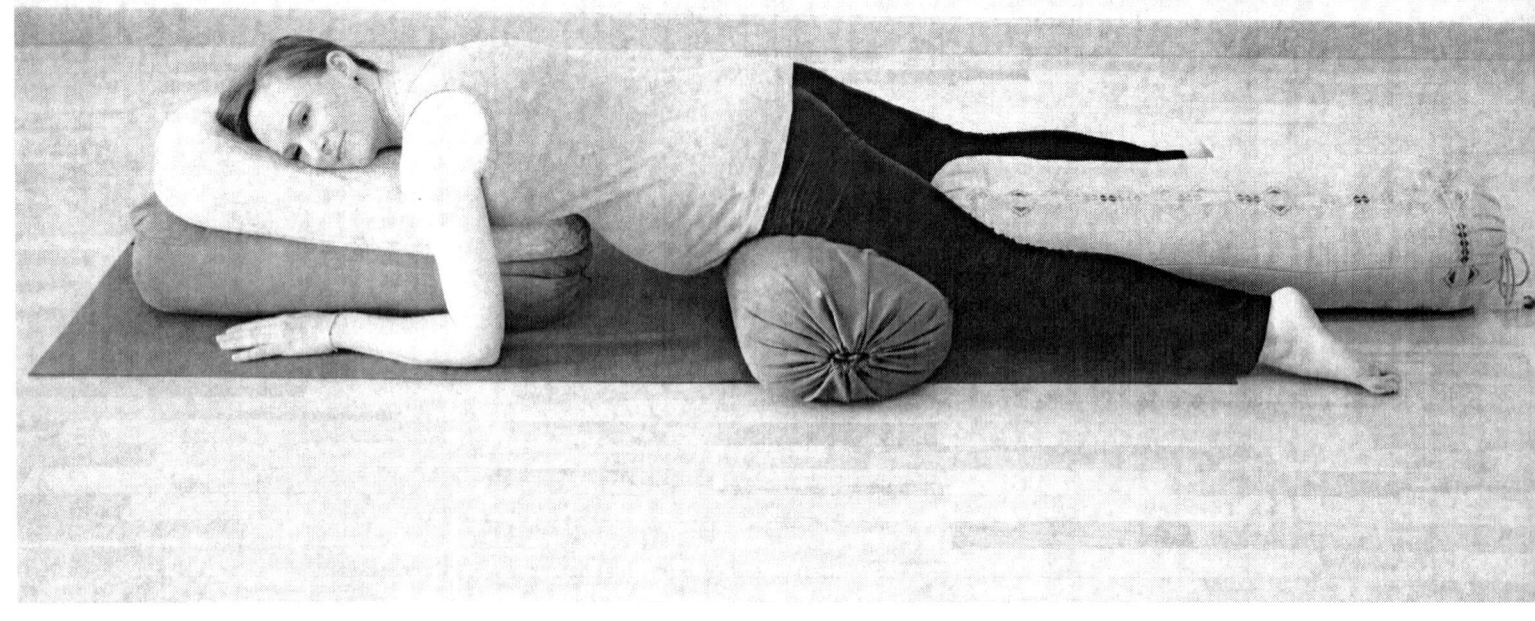

Pregnancy and Beyond: A Special Time in a Woman's Life
Getting Pregnant, Prenatal and Postnatal Postures

"Tension is who you think you should be. Relaxation is who you are." Chinese proverb

Getting Pregnant

Both men and woman can benefit from a restorative practice when trying to conceive. When a woman is trying to get pregnant, to be able to conceive she must be relaxed and open. She must become yin so the yang can enter and together create a baby. If a woman is stressed for whatever reason, be it work, family or other life issues, she must dedicate herself to learning how to relax. She needs to prepare her body to become the vessel to hold a baby. Relaxation can also be beneficial for the functioning of the male reproductive system and the ability to create healthy sperm in abundance. During the sacred space created by lovemaking and during the moments and minutes afterwards are important times to relax fully and allow the sperm to enter the egg and begin the delicate process of making a baby. In these moments bringing the insights and knowledge gained from a restorative practice can aid a couple in the process. Relaxing fully and allowing nature to work its magic in these moments can be instrumental in the conception process. An entire book can be written on the subject of conception and I am focusing here on this important relaxation practice that can be the key to unlocking the door to conceiving a baby.

As a teacher you can facilitate this understanding of relaxation and assist in the practice using the restorative sequence for getting pregnant, the postures and mind techniques given here and you can also develop your own visualizations that can aid in the conception of a baby.

Pregnancy

Both the gift of being pregnant and for almost 20 years teaching pregnant and postnatal women and their babies is such an honor and an absolute gift. There is no other time in a woman's life like this. When a woman is pregnant she becomes a vessel for spirit to manifest into form. This is a time when a woman can feel very connected to herself, the wonder of life and spirit all at the same time. Once her baby is born, the energy of the new baby here on earth, her connection with her baby and her transition process is a time to be cherished and can be approached in a way that can bring much joy, recuperation and discovery to both mom and her new baby.

The first trimester of pregnancy is a very sensitive time. Always practice with care and have students consult their health care practitioner if they have any doubts. When you plant a seed you must do all the necessary things to help it to grow. If you keep moving the soil around it from place to place it most likely won't take. You want to keep the seed that is your baby in the first trimester protected. If you have a regular practice this is not as much of an issue because you are both used to certain kinds of movements and you can move through your poses with ease. Still your first trimester needs to be taken with care, keeping the abdominal area quiet and not applying pressure or movements to the abdomen that could stress the new life that is beginning to grow inside. Throughout the pregnancy care must be taken to ensure that no deep or intense asanas that pressure the abdominal area or that put excess stress on the abdomen or the joints are practiced. The Restorative practice is generally very good throughout pregnancy when practiced with care.

In the second and third trimesters some specific variations are required to take into account your growing baby. Some poses are not recommended. With variations the practice can help to facilitate a healthy pregnancy with less stress and more ease in the delivery of your baby. As your pregnancy progresses you have the hormone relaxin flowing through your body so you need to be aware of not overstretching your joints. This hormone is there to help the pelvis open to deliver your baby so the joints become more supple. At any time during a woman's pregnancy she must always do what she is comfortable with. If for any reason your student does not feel comfortable with any posture give her an alternative or skip that one. I will explain each asana with specific information about how and when to practice it during pregnancy in the next section.

Postnatal

After having a baby your world changes. There are so many adjustments physically, mentally and practically that can be overwhelming. It can be a very tiring time for many reasons and extra rest can be hard to come by. Finding the time to rest can make a huge difference in your postnatal reality. Restorative yoga can assist you in getting the rest that you need.
After the sixth week with a vaginal birth and the tenth week with a cesarean, an active yoga practice can be resumed. The restorative postures can remain an integral part of this practice (for postnatal sequences, see pages 157 and 158).

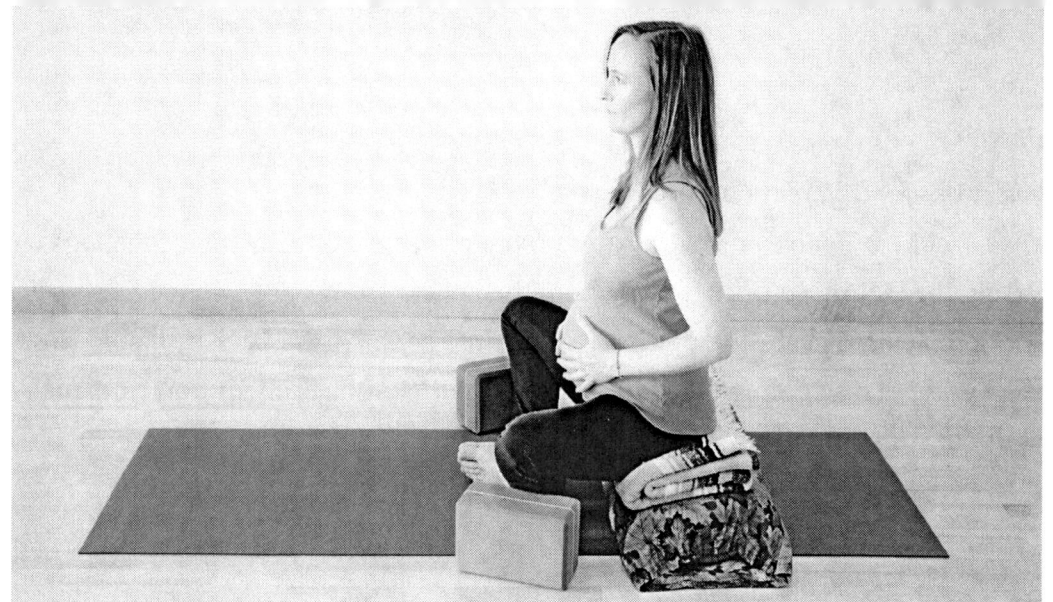

Restorative Asanas for Pregnancy

Seated and Open Legs, Forward Bends and Elongations

Supported Baddha Konasana (Supported Cobbler's Pose)

Translation
Baddha means "fixed" or "bound" and kona means "angle."

General Overview
Sometimes called the Butterfly Pose, this is a great hip and groin opener. Regular practice throughout pregnancy can help ease labor and facilitate an easy delivery.

Basic Props Needed
Two blocks or blankets for the knees and a folded blanket or pillow to support the sitting bones. For some students a wall may be needed.

Getting In and Out
Sit on the edge of your folded blanket. Bring the soles of your feet together evenly from toe to ball. Rest your knees on folded blankets, blocks or a combination of them. The height of your support is determined by the openness of your inner thighs. Support yourself with your fingertips on the floor behind you.
To come out straighten the legs on an outgoing breath. Transition to your next pose.

Benefits

Helps relieve stiffness

Opens the groins, inner thighs and knees

Stimulates the heart and abdominal organ

Improves overall circulation

Soothes sciatica

Reduces menstrual pain

Variations for Different Concerns

Knee problems: Try elevating the knees more or decrease the angle of the legs by letting the feet move further away from the pelvis.

Back problems: Elevate the pelvis, or sit against a wall if the back is unable to sit erect without discomfort. Sit against the wall with low back discomfort from pregnancy or stress.

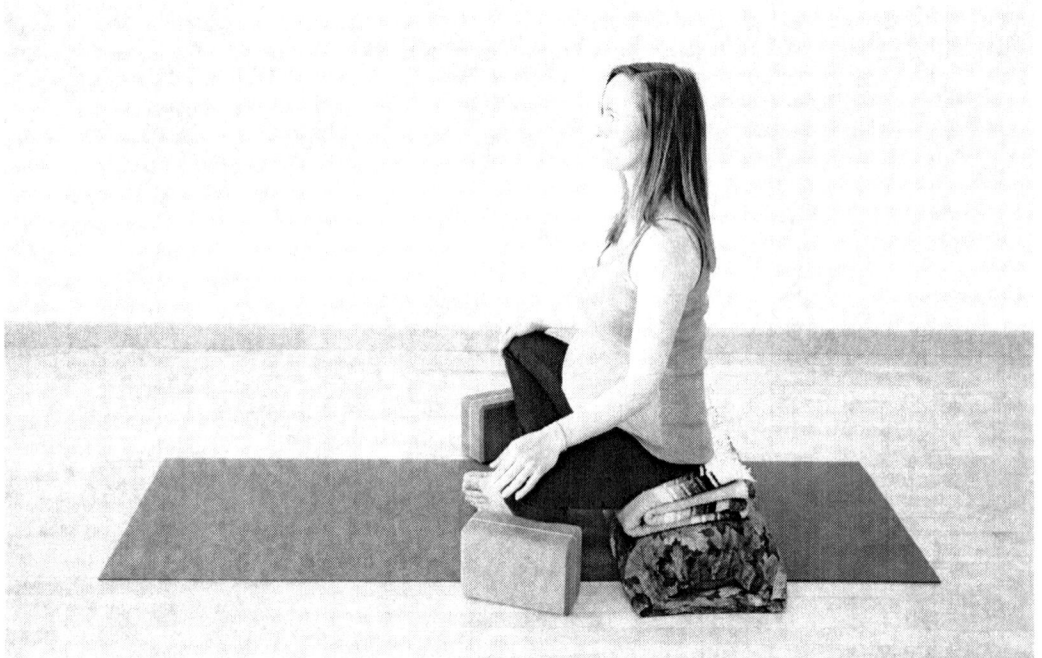

Therapeutic Application

Sciatica

Tight hips

Asthma

Flat feet

Infertility

Varicose veins

Breath in Pose

Breathe normally through the nose. Breathe into and expand the rib cage on all sides to increase the lung capacity. This is an excellent asana to practice breathing in a way that supports pregnant women. Sometimes later in pregnancy women find it difficult to breathe or to get a full deep breath; this can be because the baby is pressing on the diaphragm because of its position.

Verbal Cues

Extend the spine.

Hold the ankles and extend upward.

Press the knees down into your support, then relax.

Place your hands on the knees, press down while trying to push the knees towards each other, then relax.

Press the outside edge of your feet together and press the big toenails toward the floor, opening the feet like a book.

Externally rotate the thighs.

What to Look for With Alignment

Feet are even from toe to heel.

If one knee is supported the other also needs to be supported.

The pelvis is upright.

The back is straight.

Hands-on Assists

Root the hips down while moving your hands to lengthen from the hip creases out toward the knees.

Stand or kneel behind your student and gently pull their shoulders blades in and down the back.

Massage the shoulders with thumbs into the three points on tops of shoulders, or shoulder squeeze.

Manually open feet.

How Long to Hold the Pose

30 seconds to 3 minutes

Contraindications

In case of knee or groin injury, use a folded blanket for support under the thighs

Practice against the wall if student has asthma, bronchitis or breathlessness

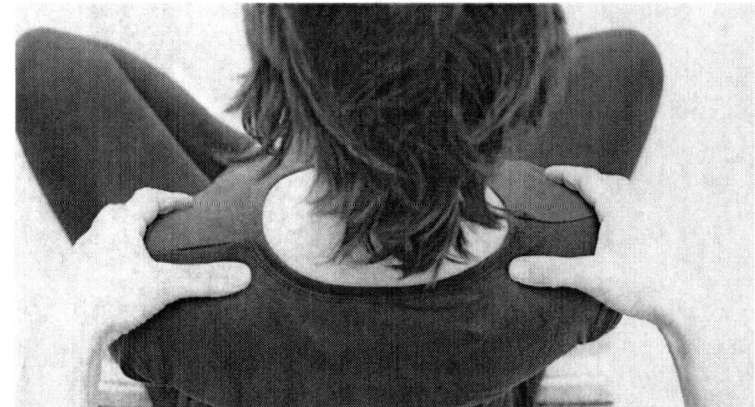

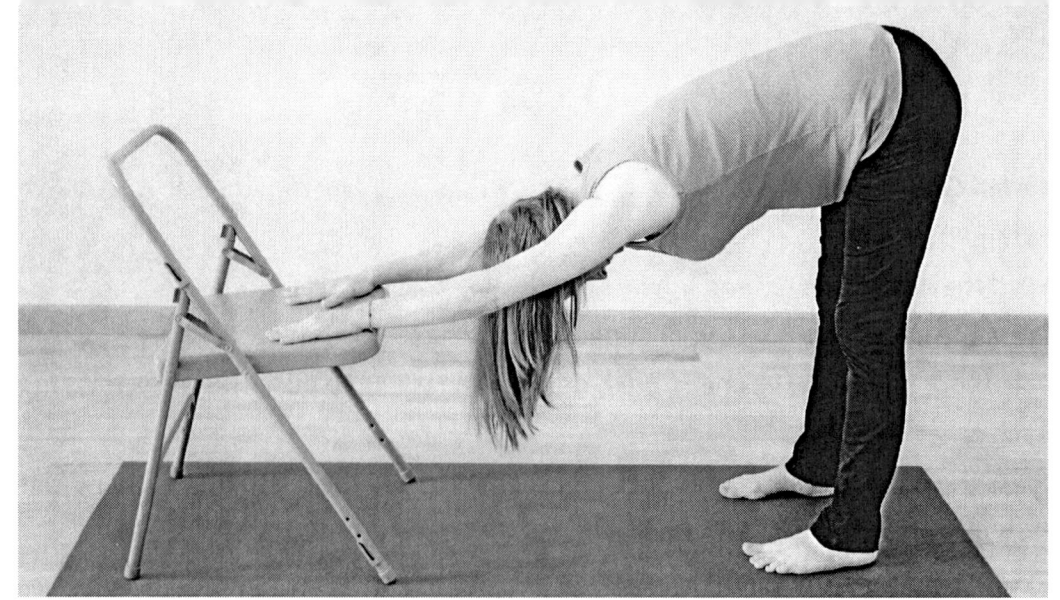

Standing Supported Uttannasana (Standing Supported Forward Bend)

Benefits

Soothes and calms the body and nervous system.

Reduces depression with regular practice

Reduces insomnia and relieves fatigue

Regulates blood pressure

Strengthens and stretches hamstrings

Increases hip joint flexibility

Strengthens knee joint and surrounding tissue and muscle

Translation

Ut means "deliberate" or "intense" and tana means "stretch," so Uttanasana is an intense forward stretch.

General Overview

This pose opens the back body while allowing support for the arms and hands, creating a sense of relaxation permitting deeper opening in a forward bend. Little by little the body releases and fuller opening happens naturally. In pregnancy the torso should always be extending and not rounding over the baby.

Basic Props Needed

Chair, several blocks or bolster combo

Getting In and Out

This asana can be done against the wall, hands resting on the wall, or in the center of the room using a chair. Stand with the feet wide enough apart so no pressure is on the belly or baby. Play with the props to get a general idea of what will be needed. Place a chair either with the front or the back of the chair facing the student depending on their flexibility. From standing position place the hands on the hips and extend upward, then keep extending as you pivot at the hips lower down and come to rest with hands or forearms resting on the support. Make sure the neck is not constricted in any way. The spine is always long and not rounding. The head can rest on the forearms if the forearms can rest comfortably on the seat of the chair.

To come out return the hands to the pelvis and extend the spine as you rise up back to standing.

Variations for Different Concerns

The hands can rest against a wall at a right angle or more (hands higher on the wall) depending on flexibility.

Therapeutic Applications

Depression
Blood pressure

Breath in Pose

Breathe normally.
Breathe into the sides of the ribcage as you extend the body.

Verbal Cues

Soften the backs of the legs. Release the back of the neck.

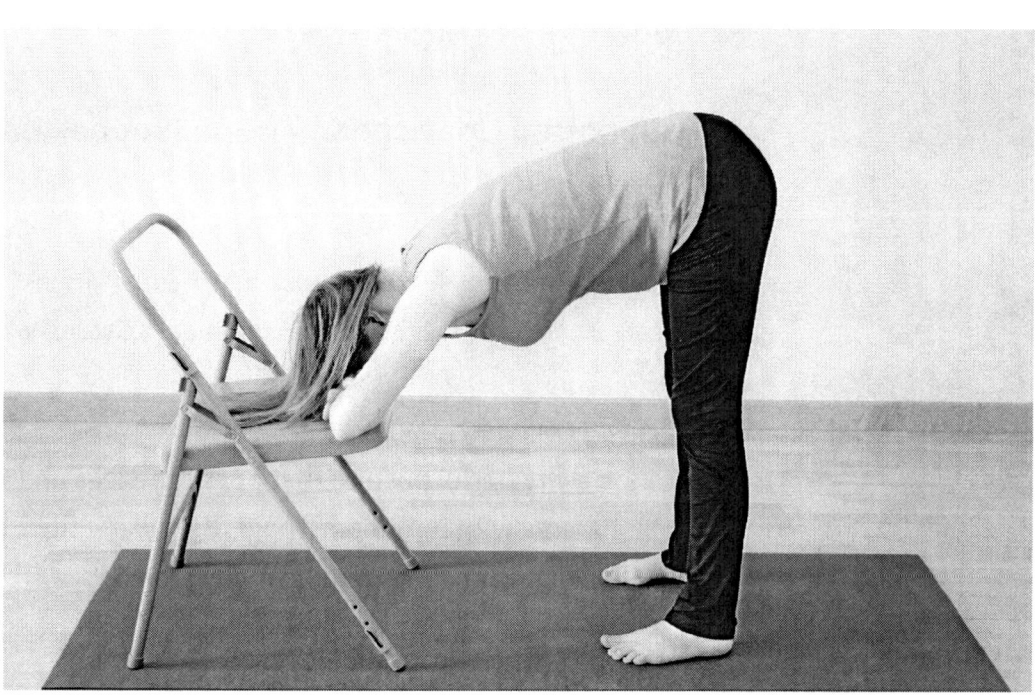

What to Look for With Alignment

Check that the torso is elongated.
As the body opens the height of the support can be lowered as long as the torso remains long and there is no pressure on the baby.
Check that the feet are wider than hip-distance apart to leave room for the baby.

Hands-on Assists

Stand behind the student and gently pull the pelvis back away from the head.

How Long to Hold the Pose

15 seconds to 1 minute

Contraindications

Osteoarthritis of the knees

Diarrhea

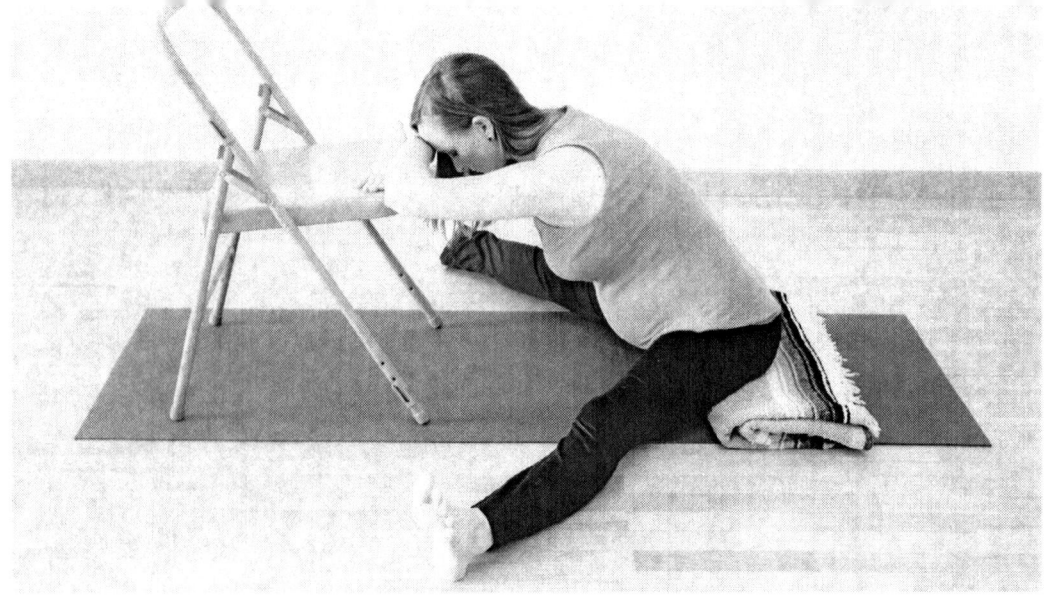

Supported Upavista Konasana (Supported Seated Wide Angle)

Translation

Upavista means "seated" and kona means "angle." Asana means "comfortable pose." Therefore Upavista Konasana means Seated Wide Angle Pose.

General Overview

This is a wonderful posture that opens the legs and releases the pelvis and back. For students with tight hamstrings, tight back, tight hips or knee problems it can be challenging and may require many props.

Basic Props Needed

A chair and one or more folded blankets

Getting In

Sit on the edge of a folded blanket, open your legs wide out to the sides with your legs straight, press out through your heels with the tips of your toes facing the ceiling. Place your chair in front of you so that your forearms can rest on the chair with the torso elongating from the pelvis to the elbows while you lean forward. Your whole torso should be lengthening. Press out through the heels stretching the legs, then relax. Breathe into the body and into the internal organs. Make sure there is no pressure on the baby.

Benefits

Helps with arthritis in the hip joints

Reduces sciatic pain

Helps prevent hernia

Massages reproductive organs

Benefits women during menstruation and pregnancy

Opens and releases hips

Opens groin muscles

Calms the brain

Getting Out
Place your hands on the chair, pull the chair closer if necessary and press up.

Variations for Different Concerns
Low back discomfort: If the low back feels sore when leaning forward decrease the forward bend using more props under the head and arms, creating less of a forward bend. Make sure the hips are elevated with a blanket or small pillow under the sitting bones, elevate higher if necessary. For some students a wall may be needed. If a student is unable to come forward at all they can work with elongating up the wall while grounding the pelvis.

Neck discomfort: The head can rest to the side, changing positions halfway through the hold time to balance the neck on both sides. If the neck is uncomfortable moving from side to side rest the forehead on the forearms so that the neck is not turned and the face is looking downward.

Inner thigh discomfort: If there is pain or strong pulling in the inner thighs bring the legs closer to each other; also make sure the pelvis is well supported.

Inner knee or back of knee discomfort: Try placing small cushions or rolled blankets under the knees, or if that does not help bring the legs closer together.

This pose can be practiced in all stages of pregnancy with varying levels of support.

Therapeutic Applications
Arthritis

Sciatica

Breath in Pose
Breathe evenly and direct the breath into the rib cage, expanding the rib cage out to the sides and breathing up into the very top of the shoulders. Breathing consciously while relaxing in the pose supports release in muscles and internal organs. It also stimulates the lymph system. As the baby gets bigger and there is less space for the internal organs, breathing into the rib cage helps to shift the focus of the breath and allow more oxygen to flow into the lungs.

Verbal Cues
Extend the spine as you move forward from the lumbar area.

Imagine the ribcage opening like a barrel, expanding on all sides at the same time with the incoming breath.

Contraindications

Lower-back injury: Sit up high on a folded blanket and keep your torso relatively upright, arms and head supported on props as the student comes forward

What to Look for With Alignment
The pelvis is supported.
There is no pressure on the baby.
The back is straight.

Hands-on Assists
Massage shoulders.
Massage down either side of the spine.
Press down on the thighs and depending on leg position roll thighs back if needed or forward.
From behind the student press the low back towards the floor.

Pregnancy
This asana can be practiced in the first and second trimesters with a chair or bolster under the chest or forehead depending on flexibility. The belly should never be crunched, the spine always elongated. There should never be any pressure on the baby/belly. In the third trimester it can be practiced with the forearms on the seat of a chair to support the body elongating and moving forward only so much as the spine is long and the belly open with no pressure of any kind on the baby, and the back is long and not rounding.

How Long to Hold the Pose
30 seconds to 2 minutes

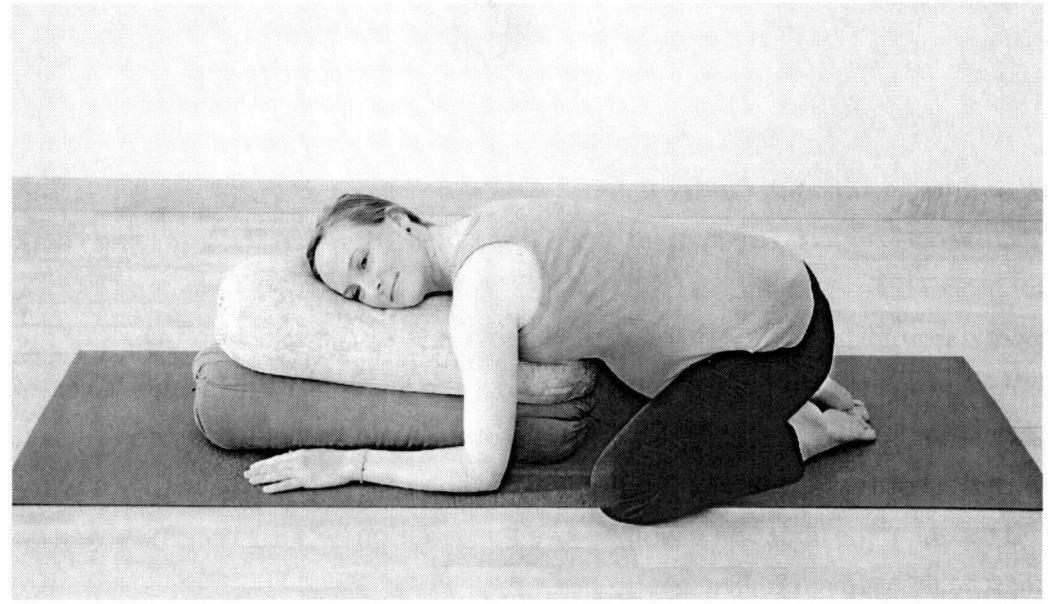

Balasana (Supported Child's Pose)

Translation
Balasana means "pose of the child."

General Overview
This asana gives a feeling of support and security and is a great counter pose to Supta Baddha

Basic Props Needed
Bolster with two blocks below (will vary with student) or two bolsters one on top of the other.

Getting In and Out
Sit on the heels and open the knees wide leaving plenty of space for your baby (see photo right). Pull the bolster and block setup in so that when you come forward only the chest rests on the bolster, leaving the belly and baby free. Place the hands on the thighs, pressing down while extending the spine upward. Lay the chest over the bolster from the sternum to the top of the head. Relax over the bolsters with the forearms resting flush to the floor and creating a right angle between the upper and lower arms.
To come out place the hands on either side of the bolster on the floor under the shoulders and press up.

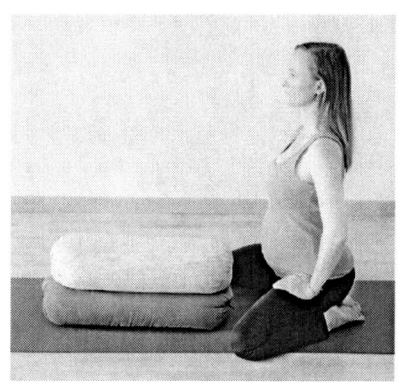

Benefits

Opens the hips, thighs, and ankles

Calms the brain

Relieves stress and fatigue

Relieves back pain

Variations for Different Concerns

Shoulder discomfort: Use support under the forearms, widen the arms and check for proper bolster height.

Knee discomfort: Place eye bags at the knee crease or use rolled-up towels or the like. You can also place something soft under the knees like a blanket or an extra sticky mat. If this does not relieve the discomfort use the legs-extended version with the bolster resting under the thighs leaving space for the belly to rest without touching the floor. Some women love this variation because they miss lying on their bellies (see photo below).

Ankle discomfort: place something below the ankle to lift up the ankle away from the floor. If this does not relieve the discomfort use the legs-extended version.

Foot discomfort: Same as for ankle.

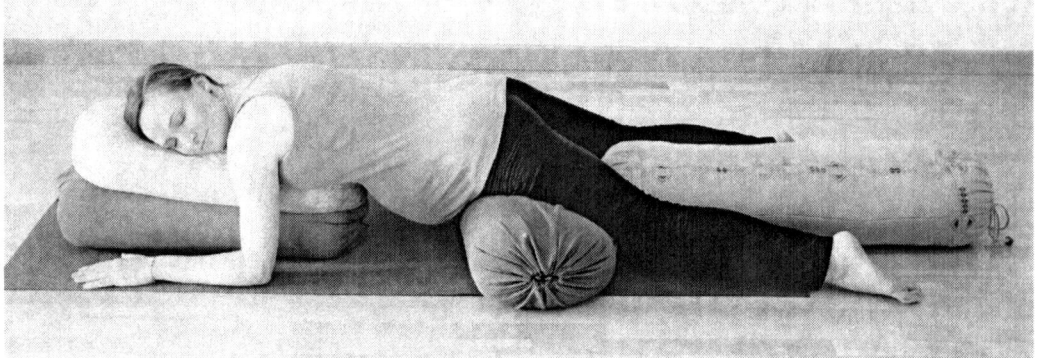

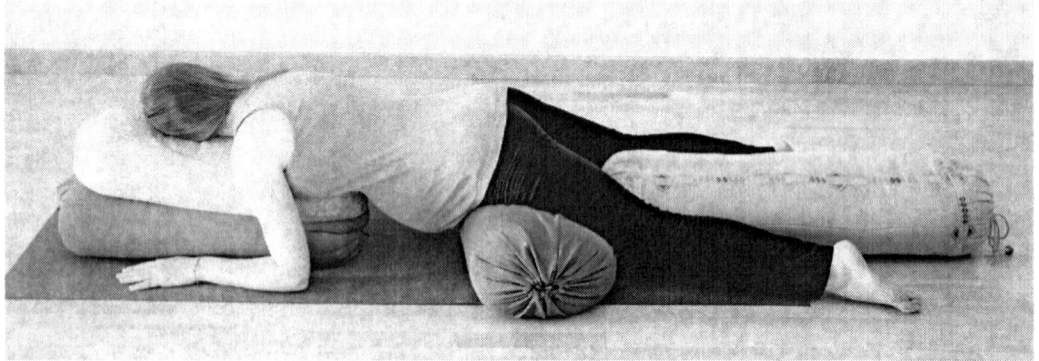

Therapeutic Applications

Stress relief

Breath in Pose

Breathe consciously into the low back, kidneys and adrenals. Breath can also be directed into the chest and rib cage.

Verbal Cues

Direct the breath focus into the back body and rib cage. Encourage the focus on feeling secure and innocent like a child.

What to Look for With Alignment

Big toes touching, knees spread wide.
Upper arm perpendicular to floor, forearms resting on the floor.
Buttocks as close to heels as in bent leg variation,

Hands-on Assists

Massage the upper back and shoulders.
Press the hands in the diagonal low back press, with the palms moving away from each other from shoulder to ileum on both sides.
Massage on either side of the spine with thumbs or palms, only where the bolster is supporting underneath.
Caution: Press gently on the low back where there is no support underneath, i.e., where the baby is.

Pregnancy

This pose can be practiced with the variation of the bolster resting under the chest, the baby resting between the bolster and the pelvis. Knees open wide.
The bolster is primarily under the chest.

How Long to Hold the Pose

1 minute to 5 minutes including head to both sides

Contraindications

Diarrhea

Knee injury (variation with legs extended)

Ankle injury (variation with legs extended)

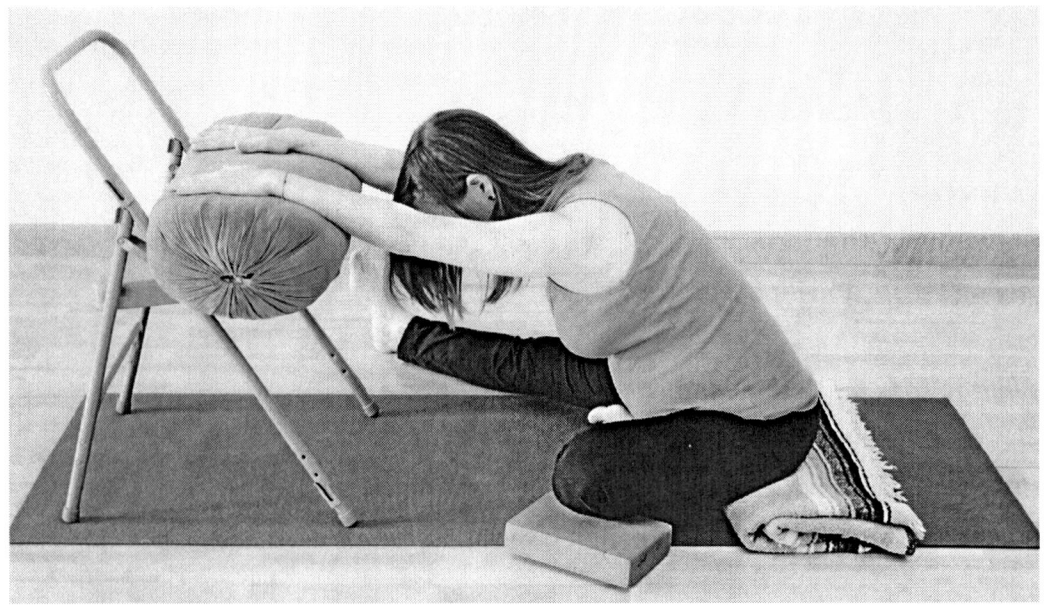

Supported Janu Sirsasana (Seated Angle Head to Knee)

Translation
Janu means "knee" and sirsa means "head."

General Overview
This is a wonderful pose to relax the nervous system. It soothes irritability and restlessness of the mind. This is a calming posture.

Basic Props Needed
Chair, blanket and block for bent leg.

Getting In and Out
Sit on the edge of a folded blanket. Open the legs creating a "v" shape between the legs so the baby can fall in the space between. Bend one leg and rest the sole of the foot on the inside of the opposite thigh. Place a bolster or blanket under the bent leg if needed. Rest your chair directly in front of you, come forward and rest your forearms then head on the chair.

Variations for Different Concerns
Back problems: Can be practiced with the back against the wall and tie around the foot.
Knee problems: Practice with support under the extended knee and/or under the bent leg knee (depending on where the issue is and how the knee feels).

Benefits

Calms the mind

Helps relieve mild depression

Elongates the spine, shoulders, hamstrings and groins

Improves digestion

Normalizes blood pressure

Improves bladder control

Relieves anxiety and fatigue

Therapeutic Applications
Stress
High blood pressure
Insomnia
Sinusitis

Breath in Pose
Breathe into both sides of the body fully and evenly. Expand the rib cage outward with your inhalation and relax with the exhalation, then breathe normally. Breathe into the back of the extended leg.

Verbal Cues
Relax the shoulders, relax the face.
Make sure there is no pressure on your baby.
Keep the spine elongating.

What to Look for With Alignment
Reach both arms evenly forward to support the torso and rest the forearms then the forehead on the edge of the seat of the chair. The movement of the torso is directly forward between the legs.

Hands-on Assists
Stand or kneel behind the student, facing their back. Place your hands against their lower back and pelvis. The hands should be turned so the fingers point towards the tailbone. The pressure isn't to push them deeper into the forward bend; rather, gentle pressure (parallel to the line of the back in a downward direction towards the tailbone in line with the spine) encourages the spine and tailbone to lengthen away from the torso, ground them and release the back gently.
Massage the shoulders.
Adjust the student's body gently and encourage extension, moving hands or thumbs gently along either side of the spine from the pelvis to the shoulders, encouraging length not pressing the body further forward.

Pregnancy
Instead of resting over the leg, rest directly forward in the center of both legs. This pose can be practiced coming forward and resting the head on the back of the

Contraindications

Asthma

Diarrhea

Acute knee injury

hands and the forearms on the seat of a chair and keeping the spine long. Always keep the belly open without folding over it or creating any pressure on the abdomen, leaving plenty of space for baby.

How Long to Hold the Pose
30 seconds to 3 minutes per side

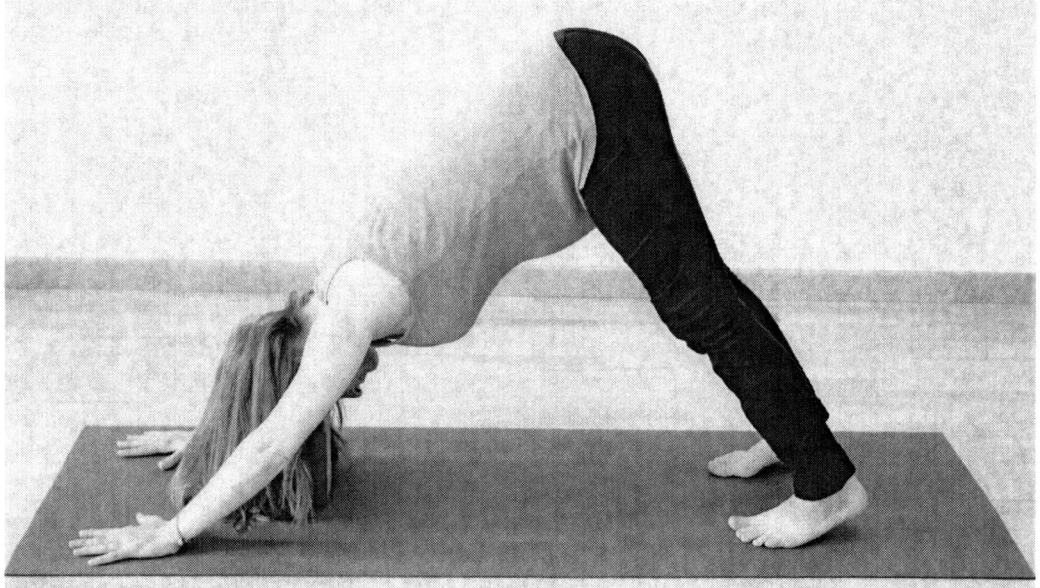

Adho Mukha Svanasana (Downward-Facing Dog)

Translation
Adho means "facing down" and svan means "dog."

General Overview
This is the multivitamin asana of yoga which opens and strengthens the body; it is an excellent pose for opening the hamstrings, back, shoulders and hands while bringing strength to the arms, wrists, hands and torso. Some practitioners consider this asana an inversion and for a pregnant woman it can feel like that so go slowiy and women can rest in Child's Pose at any time.

Basic Props Needed
Mat, block(s) or bolster and a wall for three variations

Getting In
From Child's Pose with wide legs extend the arms out on the floor. Do not change the hand distance or position, plant the hands and come to Table Pose. Make sure the hands are well connected to the earth. The middle fingers are parallel, hands plugged into the earth like a plug into a socket, all the skin of the hand is touching the mat and the fingers are comfortably apart. Tuck the toes under and extend the legs and lift the tailbone upward toward the sky. Adjust the block or bolster so the forehead can rest on it without any bending of the arms to reach it.

Restorative Yoga

Benefits

Calms the brain

Helps relieve stress

Relieves mild depression

Energizes the body

Opens the shoulders, hamstrings, calves, arches and hands

Strengthens the arms and legs and arches of the feet

Helps prevent osteoporosis

Improves digestion

Relieves headache

Relieves insomnia

Relieves back pain

Relieves fatigue

Getting Out
To come out, bend the legs at the knees, open the knees wide and bring the knees to the mat. Rest in wide leg Child's Pose. Place hands under shoulders and come out.

Variations for Different Concerns
Fingers going up the wall, head on block for arthritis, stiff shoulders, elbows or hands.

Heels on the wall, forehead resting on a block, good for relieving cramps in the calf muscles, strengthening calves and arches in the feet.

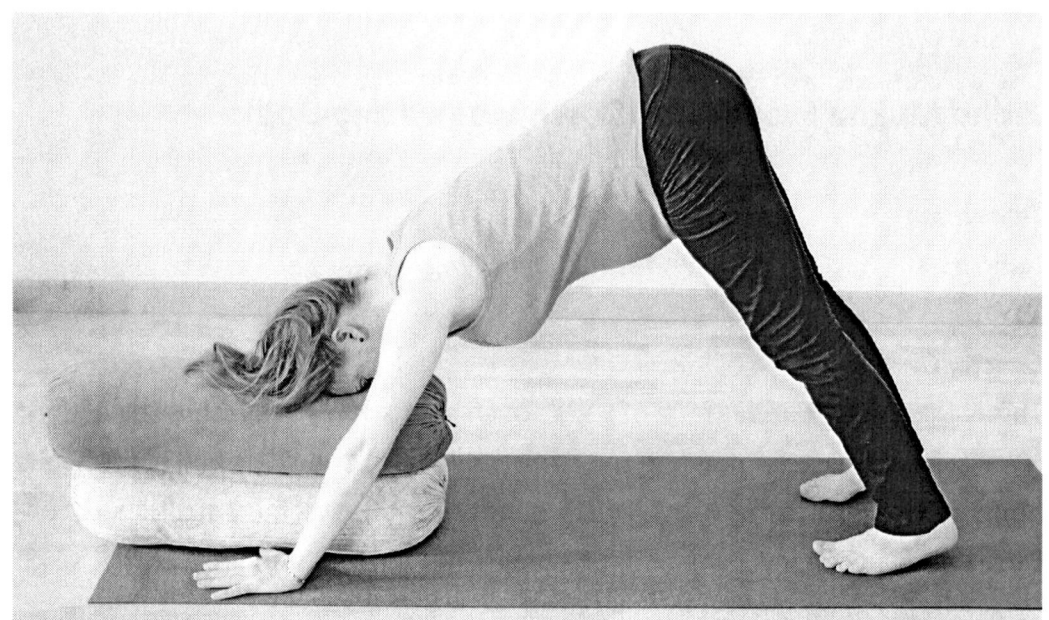

Therapeutic Applications
High blood pressure

Asthma

Flat feet

Sciatica

Sinusitis

Breath in Pose
Breathe normally through the nose.

Verbal Cues
Press the thighs, knees and ankles back in the direction of the wall behind you.

Press the hands completely into the floor; there should be no space between the skin of the hands and the floor. Rest the head and neck fully.

What to Look for With Alignment
When resting the head on a bolster or block be sure the student is not bending their arms to reach the block but opening the body enough, feet and hands away from each other, to allow the head to reach the support. Sometimes more support is needed under the forehead.
If possible the arms should rest by the ears.

Hands-on Assists
Press the low back pelvis towards the coccyx.

Pregnancy
Practice with shorter holding times, especially at the end of the third trimester, as is comfortable. When getting in and out always make sure there is plenty of room for the baby.

How Long to Hold the Pose
3 to 30 seconds

Contraindications

Carpal tunnel syndrome

Diarrhea

Varicose veins

High blood pressure or headache: The head must be supported on a bolster or block.

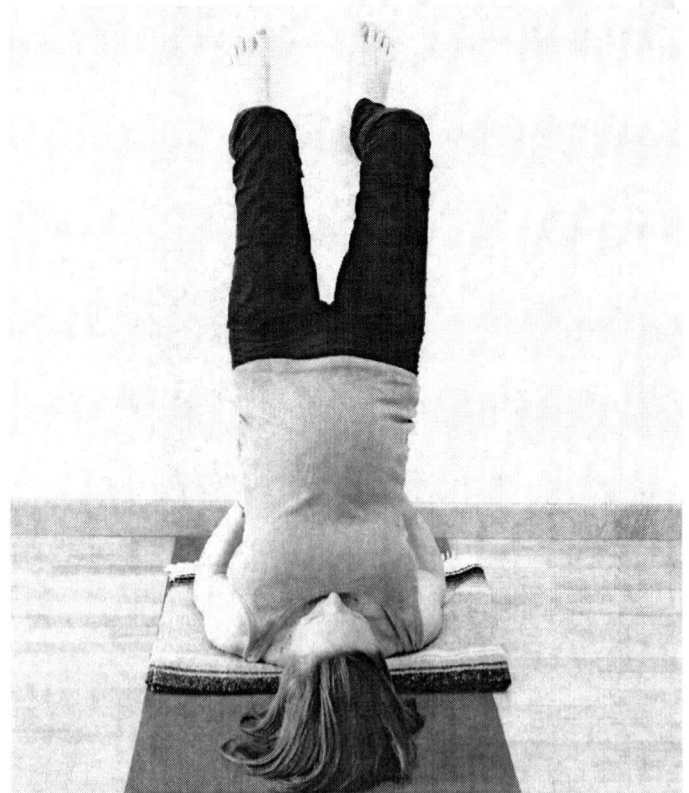

Pregnancy Inversion

Supported Salamba Sarvangasana (Supported Shoulder Stand)

Translation
Salamba means "propped up" and sarvanga means "all the limbs," so we have "all the limbs propped up."

General Overview
This classic asana is referred to as the "Queen of the asanas" while Sirsasana (Head Stand) is referred to as the king. Sarvangasana cultivates feminine yin energy and has so many wonderful benefits.

Basic Props Needed
A wall and a mat (blanket for shoulders if legs come off wall)

Getting In and Out
The challenge of this pose can be getting into the pose. You want to get your buttocks as close to the wall as possible. Lie down on your side with your buttocks touching the wall. This can be challenging with a big belly. One you are as close into the wall as possible open the legs and swing the legs up the wall, place the feet onto the wall and lift the pelvis towards the center of the room taking the

Contraindications

Diarrhea

Headache

High blood pressure

Neck injury

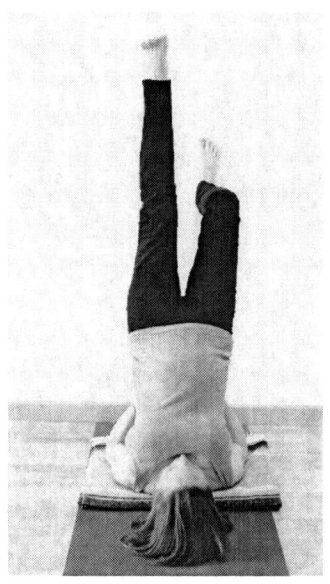 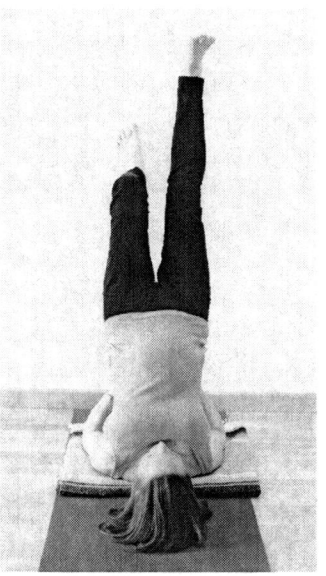 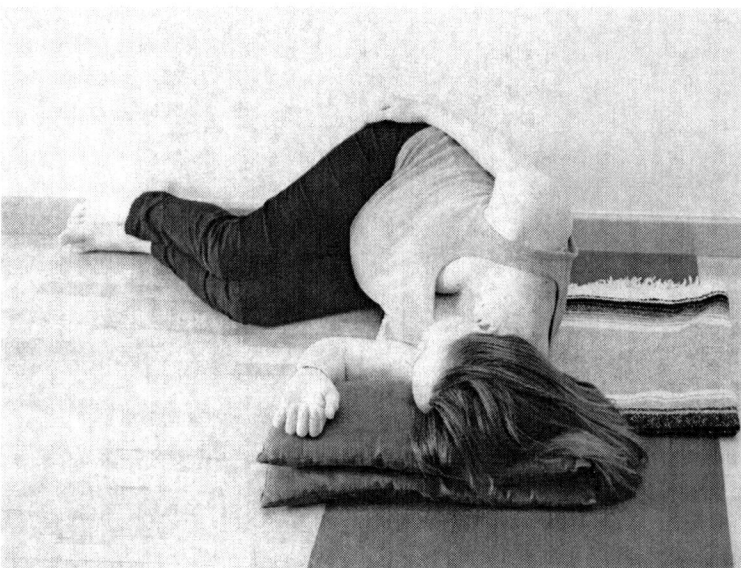

pressure off of the vena cava immediately.

Keep the feet at the level of the knees. After you lift from the wall interlace the fingers under the body and bring the elbows in towards each other, then release the fingers and place the hands on the low back, thumbs to the outside, fingers facing upward towards the feet. Lift one foot at a time towards the ceiling for two to four breaths then return the leg to the wall and lift the opposite foot up.

To come out, release the hands slowly, lower the pelvis down and roll to the left side; support the head on a block or cushion and rest. When you feel the blood has settled gradually come up.

Therapeutic Applications

Asthma

Sinusitis

Swollen legs ankles and feet

I have had students practice this pose to try to get their babies to turn head down, but it is difficult to determine whether it helped or not.

Breath in Pose

Breathe normally through the nose.

Verbal Cues

Feel the energy running down the legs.

Sense the thyroid gland being washed with blood and fresh energy.

Press the back of the head gently into the floor.

Benefits

Calms the brain

Relieve stress and mild depression

Stimulates the thyroid gland

Stimulates abdominal organs

Lengthens the shoulders and neck

Tones the legs and buttocks

Alleviates swelling in legs and feet

Improves digestion

Reduces fatigue

Benefits

Alleviates insomnia

Alleviates hypertension

Soothes the nervous system

Alleviates urinary problems

Beneficial for varicose veins

Supports circulatory system

Improves bowel movements and relieves colitis

Alleviates asthma, bronchitis and throat ailments

Give plenty of assurance to come out of the pose at any time discomfort is felt.

What to Look for With Alignment
Check the neck and head for alignment. Check that the elbows are in alignment with the shoulders.
Check that there is space between the chin and chest. The chest can press toward the chin and the back of the head can press towards the floor.

Hands-on Assists
Bring the elbows in if they are splayed out.
If there is swelling in the feet, ankles and/or legs: When inverted bring your hands to the leg at the ankle and allow the full hand, fingers and palms to contact the leg. From ankle towards the heart gently massage creating a kind of cylinder with your two hands and fingers down the leg to just below the knee. You can repeat this stroke several times.

Pregnancy
If you are experienced with this pose, you can continue to practice it late into pregnancy. I suggest the version keeping at least one leg on the wall for pregnant woman in the second and third trimesters. The legs can be elevated one leg at a time for 2-4 breaths on each side. If any discomfort is felt come down immediately and rest on your left side with support under the head until the blood has normalized. This pose can be practiced throughout the three trimesters. Careful attention must be paid in the third trimester. Never practice if discomfort is felt. Because of the extra blood supply in the body during pregnancy pressure can be felt in the head. The weight of the baby can also press up into the lungs and stomach and can cause discomfort. If the student is uncomfortable at any time have them come down and rest on their left side, head supported. Do not rest at all on the back in the second and third trimesters; from a side-lying position go to the back and then directly up into the shoulder stand, lifting the pelvis up swiftly. Great pose for ankle swelling with massage assist on ankles and calves. When coming out roll immediately off to the left side, support the head and rest before sitting up.

How Long to Hold the Pose
5 seconds to 4 minutes

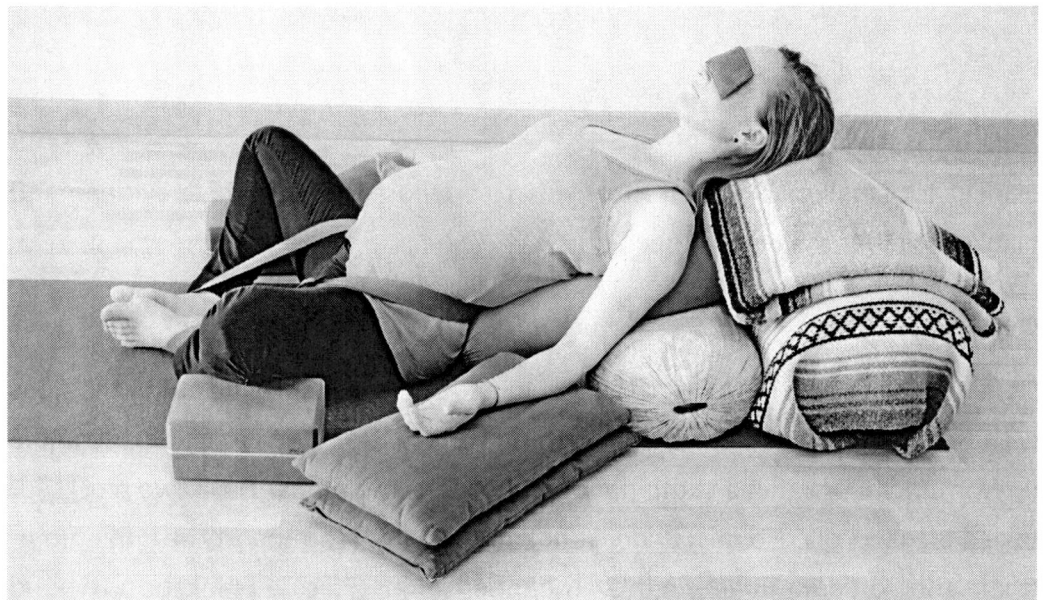

Supine (Lying Back) and Side Lying

A note on supine postures: During pregnancy the vena cava is a vein that supports the baby. Anatomically, it lies just to the right of the midline--just on the right side of the spine. As the baby gets bigger, the uterus becomes heavier; lying flat on the vena cava will (like stepping on a garden hose) obstruct flow up towards the heart. The return of blood from the lower half of the body becomes sluggish, which can increases the swelling of your ankles, feet and legs, can cause dizziness and can have an impact on hemorrhoids as well. This is why it is not recommended to lie on your back during pregnancy. Take this into consideration with all your yoga poses when working with pregnant women.

Supta Baddha Konasana (Reclining Bound Angle Pose)

Translation
Supta means "reclining," baddha means "fixed" or "bound" and kona means "angle."

General Overview
This is one of the most popular restorative postures for pregnant women. Enjoyed by almost all students with variations to accommodate individual concerns. Next to Savasana it is the most widely practiced restorative posture. Pregnant women love this pose as it gives a sense of lying back and feels so good to open the front of the body.

Basic Props Needed
Two or more bolsters, two blocks (or two blankets or two cushions), one folded

Benefits

Regulates blood pressure

Soothes and tones the digestive system

Tones the kidneys

Improves blood circulation in the ovary area

Relieves varicose veins

Relieves sciatica

Helps correct a prolapsed uterus

Reduces the pain caused by hemorrhoids

Softens hips and groins

Helps to alleviate depression

Helps to relieve anxiety

Opens the chest

---

blanket (or small pillow), extra blankets to support the arms, belt, eye bag and blanket to cover the body (if needed).

Getting In

Sit in Baddha Konasana, soles of the feet joined and knees splaying out to the sides with the short end of your bolsters behind you creating a 30- to 45-degree angle up from the floor using a combination of bolsters and props. Have two blocks (or folded blankets or cushions) under your knees, enough to support the inner groin--there should be no pulling felt on the inner thighs. Place a blanket on the end of your bolster to rest your head on. Make a loop in your belt and place the belt around your body on the low back sacral area and along the inside of your knees, then around and under your feet. Place blankets at the sides to support the arms. Using your hands and arms to help you, slowly lie back onto the bolsters and props. Adjust the blanket to rest under your head. Place the eye bag over the eyes.

Getting Out

To come out of the pose, place your hands palms down on the floor, and in one movement using your hands to support you lift your head in the direction of your chest and sit up. Use the arms and hands pressing into the floor to help you to sit up, not the abdominal muscles.

*Note that the abdominal muscles cannot be strained during pregnancy. When going down into the pose, with the support of the arms the abdominal muscles can be engaged lightly. When coming out of the pose the abdominal muscles should remain completely passive, the arms do all the work.

Variations for Different Concerns

Low back discomfort: Move the feet out several inches away from the body.
Adjust the neck (head level).
Raise the level of the bolster even more.
Move the bolster(s) out away from the pelvis.
Shoulder discomfort: Place additional folded blankets or small pillows under the arms.
Turn the palms down.
Neck discomfort: Make sure the head is fully supported and check the angle of the head and neck for alignment. Work with adjusting the head level until the student is comfortable. The throat should be soft and relaxed.

Inner thigh or groin discomfort: Make sure the inner thighs are fully supported by placing more support under the bent legs. If this doesn't remedy the situation extend the legs out and rest them flat on the floor or with the knees over a bolster and the feet resting on the floor or on blocks or some prop if the feet don't reach the floor easily.

Knee discomfort: Depending on the level of discomfort and mobility. First try using more support under the knees; if this does not alleviate the discomfort allow the legs to rest forward with a bolster under the knees.

Therapeutic Applications

Stress and anxiety

Depression

Opening the front of the body

Digestion

Opening the heart

Regulation of blood pressure

Breath in Pose

I will often guide students to breathe into their chests and expand the upper body while this area is being accentuated by the bolsters. For pregnant women this is particularly helpful as their breathing can be affected by their growing baby. Sometimes during pregnancy in the second and more in the third trimester women experience trouble breathing. At times the baby can push up against the diaphragm and cause pressure on the lungs. This is an excellent time to practice breathing out into the rib cage and expanding the upper area of the lungs. During the inhalation allow the ribs in the front to expand out with the inhalation, exhale slowly, on the next breath allow the ribcage to expand out to the sides and up into the armpits, exhaling slowly. On the third inhalation expand the ribcage out in the back of the body. On the forth breath expand all sides of the torso like you are breathing into a wine barrel that expands on all sides with the inhalation and contracts gently with the exhalation. Breath for four breaths expanding out on all sides of the rib cage. Stay fully relaxed while practicing. When not focusing on any particular way of breathing the breath is soft and natural through the nose. Never strain when doing pranayama; if you feel out of breath or strained in any way resume breathing normally.

Contraindications

If you have spondylolisthesis, spondylolysis or diagnosed disc disease

If there is pain in the back that cannot be remedied by variations

After 3 months of pregnancy must practice with variation

Verbal Cues

Bring your shoulder blades together and onto your back, then relax.

Take your hands to the flesh of your buttocks and slide the flesh towards your feet, opening a space in your low back.

Visualize a bud of a flower in your heart chakra and see it opening up into full bloom, one petal at a time, or slowly opening all the petals at once.

Feel your baby being nourished while you rest in this position.

What to Look for With Alignment

Make sure the bolsters are straight behind your student.

Make sure their feet are even big toe to heel.

Make sure the strap is in the correct place on the sacral part of the back and looped correctly.

Look for an even angular line from forehead to nose, to chest to belly, to feet, going from up to down evenly.

Make sure their body is in a line, head to shoulders, shoulders to pelvis and pelvis to feet.

Make sure there is no discomfort anywhere in the body.

Hands-on Assists

Moving the shoulder blades, in and down: Flattening and releasing the shoulders and shoulder blades. This is done by inviting the student to relax completely then sliding the hands under the shoulder blades and directing them in and down. A massage may be given to the rhomboids (the muscles located between the shoulder blades and spine) with the fingertips when hands are under the shoulders.

Thumbs in three points in shoulders: Press the thumbs into the tops of the shoulders starting close to the neck and moving out towards the arms.

Gentle neck pull: Hold the head with hands, fingertips under the occipital ridge (where the head meets the neck), and pull the head towards you gently.

Head hold: Hold the head and encourage deep relaxation of the head into the hands.

Occipital ridge release: Place the fingers on the neck just below the occipital ridge and allow the student's head to rest in your hands and their neck to soften into your fingers.

Heart to neck or head polarity: Lay one hand on the heart and one hand under the neck.

Hand massage: Giving a simple hand massage while your student is resting can be a powerful way to encourage deeper relaxation.

Arm swing: Taking your student's wrist and lifting their arm, gently swing the arm back and forth. If they are not fully relaxed you will feel them holding their arm. Encourage them to let go and to make their arm heavy. If they are unable to relax their arm take the elbow and wrist, supporting their arm more fully with small gentle movements continue to encourage them to let go. Then gently release their arm back to the earth. Often they will be able to surrender and relax, but if they are not able simply encourage them to continue to be aware and to practice relaxation.

Foot massage: (when legs are extended) With pregnant women do not massage the kidney point in the center of the sole of the foot and do not massage the ankles with any depth; pressing points on the ankle can stimulate contractions.

Aura circle around heart: With the hands about 5 or 6 inches above the heart with the palms facing towards your student's body, make a circle in the air creating the shape of a circle above and around their heart center which is in the center of the chest. Allow each hand to make a circle in an inward direction: The right hand will circle from right to left and the left hand will circle from left to right. The circles will overlap each other over the student's heart center.

Pregnancy

In second and third trimesters the pose can be modified to create an angle that keeps the womb from pressing on the vena cava (the major vein that brings blood to the baby), which runs along the inside of the spine on the right side. Extra support is needed under the arms as well as for the back.

How Long to Hold the Pose

2 to 30 minutes

Benefits

Opens the abdomen

Strengthens the arches

Helps correct flat feet

Relieves tired legs

Improves digestion

Helps prevent arterial blockages

Increases the elasticity of lung tissue

Enhances resistance to infections

Relieves indigestion, acidity and flatulence

Corrects a prolapsed uterus, and tones the pelvic organs

Elongates the thighs and deep hip flexors (psoas), knees and ankles.

Reduces inflammation in the knees, and relieves gout and rheumatic pain

Relieves pain and fatigue in the legs and feet, alleviating the effects of long hours of standing

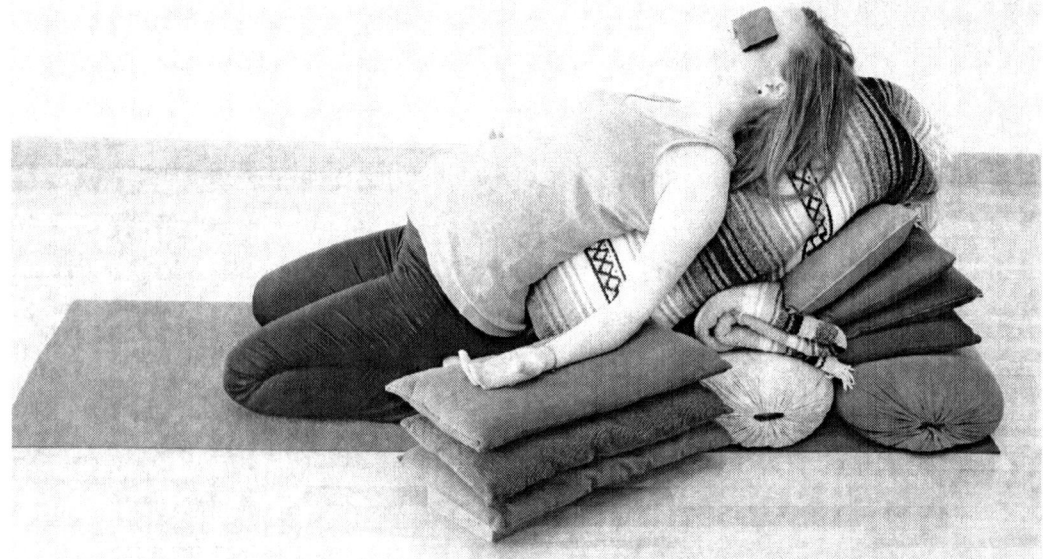

Supta Virasana (Reclining Hero Pose)

Translation
Supta means "lying down" and vira means "hero" or "champion."

General Overview
This is a beneficial posture that can be challenging for some students. With patience and understanding of how to practice with the support of props, it can be practiced by many and the benefits are plentiful.

Basic Props Needed
Bolsters, blankets and often block(s) and eye bag(s).

Getting In and Out
Determine how much support is needed to sit with comfort in Virasana. With that amount of support under the pelvis and possibly a bit more depending on the openness of the quadriceps, build up the support behind the student with bolsters and other props so that they can lie back without discomfort and with support in no less than a 45-degree angle. Place something under the forearms as shown in the photo to create support for the shoulders. Slowly lie back using the arms for support.

To come out use the arms to help, pressing the hands into the floor as you bring the chin towards the chest and sit up in one smooth movement. Avoid engaging the abdominal muscles to come up.

Variations for Different Concerns

This pose may require many props to create comfort for your student. Some students will not be able to practice this asana, particularly if they have very tight quadriceps.

Knee and ankle discomfort: Place a block or two as needed under the pelvis, equally raise the height of the bolsters to be even with the pelvic support and then from there raise the bolster to a 30- to 45-degree angle to support the back fully.

Low back discomfort: Raise the bolster(s) to create a greater angle when lying back. Tuck the tailbone forward.

Knee discomfort: Place an eye bag or small rolled towel in the back of the knee. Depending on where the discomfort lies, a blanket or small cushion can be placed under the knees.

Therapeutic Applications

Arthritis

Asthma

Digestive roblems

Flat feet

Headache

High blood pressure

Insomnia

Respiratory ailments

Sciatica

Varicose veins

Knee problems

Breath in Pose

Breathe into the front of the body and into the rib cage and lungs.
Breathe gently and normally.

Verbal Cues

Feel the front of the body opening.
Relax the thighs.

What to Look for With Alignment

Check for the bolster being aligned under the body.

Contraindications

If there are any serious back, knee or ankle problems, or pain in the knees, ankles, feet or low back that cannot be remedied by variations to support these areas avoid this pose

Do not practice if there are problems with a heart condition

Check for the angle of support from the lower to the upper ends of the body.
Check for the foot position on both sides, toenails touching the floor, heels facing upwards towards the sky at the outside of the thighs.
Check for feet resting at the sides of the thighs, not under.
Check that the thighs are parallel to each other in the first trimester. In the second and third trimesters, when the baby is bigger, the thighs may be allowed to open away from each other creating space for the baby if it is necessary. Check that the arms are well supported so there is no hanging in the shoulders.

Hands-on Assists
Head hold, gentle neck pull
Shoulder press, and thumbs into the three points in tops of the shoulders
Hand massage

Pregnancy
In second and third trimesters this pose can be modified to create an angle of 30- to 45-degrees that keeps the womb from pressing on the vena cava (the major vein that brings blood to the baby) which runs along the inside of the spine on the right side. This pose needs to be practiced with extra props to allow the upper body to be supported more fully, blankets or cushions under the arms and extra support for the head as needed. Legs can be open, hands can rest palms down. Make sure the arms are supported and not hanging in any way. There should be no pain of any kind while practicing this or any pose during pregnancy.

How Long to Hold the Pose
10 seconds to 10 minutes

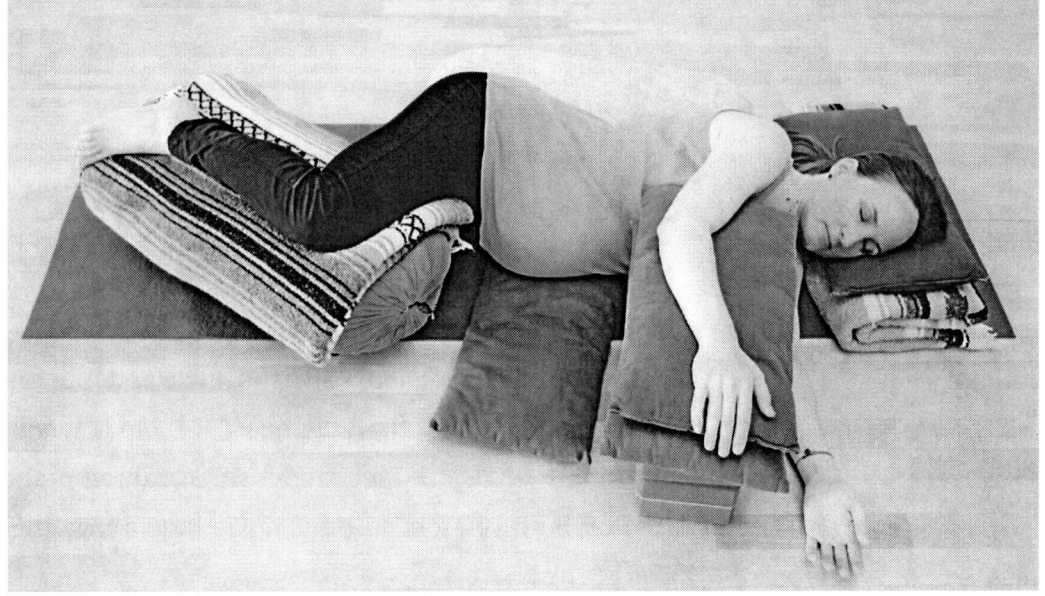

Savasana (Corpse Pose)

Translation
Sava means "corpse."

General Overview
This is one of the most basic and important restorative poses that can be modified for pregnancy. Deep relaxation can be achieved and many benefits can be gained.

Basic Props Needed
Head support.
Bolster or rolled blanket(s) between the legs.
Small folded blanket or small cushion under belly in second and third trimesters.
Bolster or rolled blanket for the back especially if there is back pain.
Bolster or cushions for the upper arm.
Blanket for cover if needed.

Getting In and Out
Gather your props and place them close to where they will eventually go. Lie down on your left side with support under the head, between the legs, support under belly (baby) and support for the upper arm. If needed, back support is also recommended.

Benefits

Calms the brain and relieves stress and mild depression

Relaxes the body

Reduces headache, fatigue and insomnia

Helps to regulate blood pressure.

Promotes inner peace and tranquility

Improves memory and concentration

Supports immune system function

Soothes the nervous system

Improves circulation to and function of organs and organ systems

Alleviates discomforts associated with pregnancy

Restorative Yoga

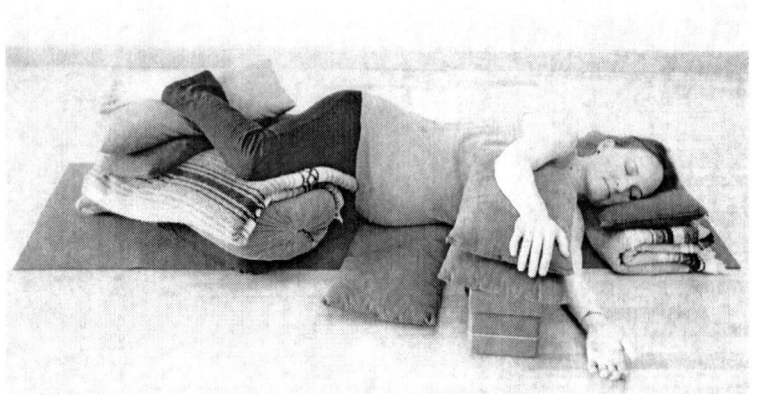

Variations for Different Concerns
Foot, ankle or leg swelling: Raise the ankle and foot on the higher leg higher than the heart. If there is swelling in both ankles or feet, the position can be practiced on both sides, raising the ankle high above the level of the heart.

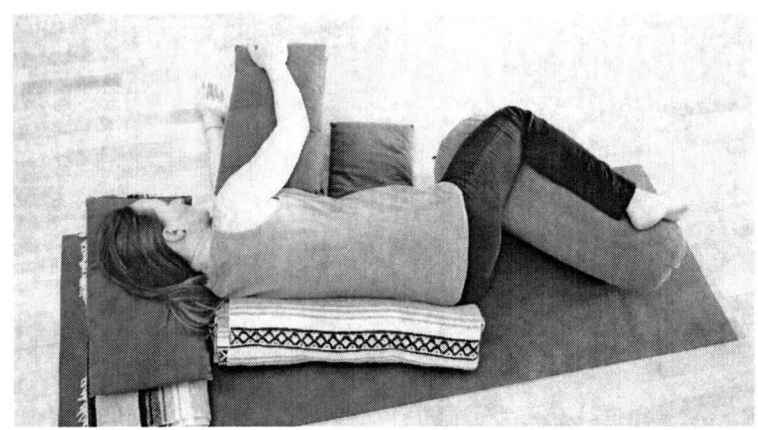

Low back discomfort: Offer support for the back by placing a bolster or folded blankets behind the entire back, particularly the low back. Support the belly as this will relieve the pulling on the back.

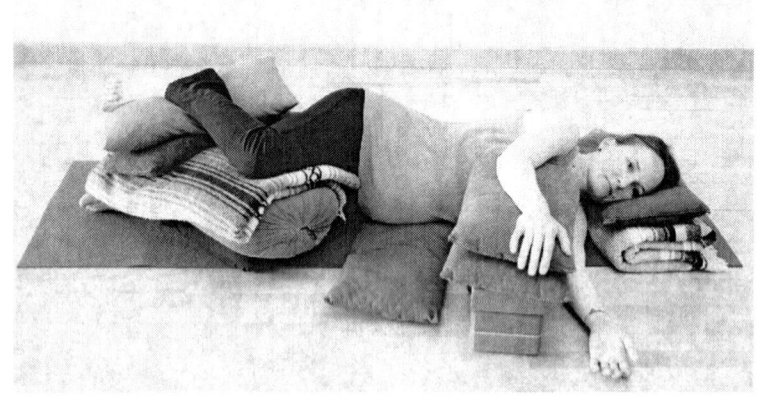

Hip discomfort: Place support for the legs from the mid thigh down to and including the feet. Make sure the legs are pelvis-width apart.

Therapeutic Applications
Stress
Depression
Recovery from illness
Anxiety

Breath in Pose
Normal gentle breath

Verbal Cues

This pose can be led with a progressive relaxation.
It is powerful for moms to visualize their babies at the developmental stage they are at and send loving kindness to their babies.

What to Look for With Alignment

Look for the legs to be bent so that the soles of the feet are even with the back. Look for the support in the upper arm so that the upper arm rests parallel to the floor creating plenty of space for the chest. See that the belly is supported correctly and that the back is supported.

Hands-on Assists

Assist your student in becoming comfortable, checking and adjusting props so that they are fully supported and able to let go.

How Long to Hold the Pose

2 to 30 minutes

Contraindications

Variation for pregnancy, side lying with support

CHAPTER 12

Sequencing for Your Class or Individual Students

"Every now and then go away, have a little relaxation, for when you come back to your work your judgment will be surer."
Leonardo DaVinci

In your sequencing, look to open particular parts of the body (or several areas) or address a mental state or illness through a variety of positions. Depending on the time that you have, and the areas that you wish to address, adjust your sequence.

When sequencing for specific conditions consider as many aspects of your student or students that you can. Research the benefits and contraindications. Consider the abilities of your student(s)--with this information you can create your own sequence.

You can also place one restorative pose at the beginning or end of a more active class as part of your class sequence.

Working with Specific Conditions

There are many postures that address stress and so many that can address so many different ailments. You can create your own series to address specific concerns based on the benefits and contraindications of the asanas, keeping in mind a balance of forward and backward postures, inverted and twisting to create a correct balance for your students. This is not to say that you need to include all four types in each sequence. The following are some sequences that I have used for the conditions listed below. Sequences can also always be simplified--sometimes less is more and spending more time in each posture with fewer postures in the practice can work very well.

I have included time suggestions for the poses. These times can be adjusted as needed.

Sequence for Getting Pregnant, Pre-Pregnancy

This sequence requires a mental focus on becoming receptive and an understanding of how to relax the body and calm the mind. Use the visualizations from Chapter 7 and other techniques to help the student to relax fully and become receptive.

Warm-up Series with a focus on the pelvis and ovary area, 10-20 minutes (page 32)

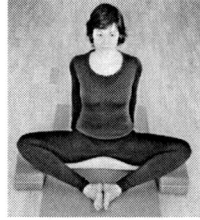

Supported Baddha Konasana
(page 63)
1 to 3 minutes

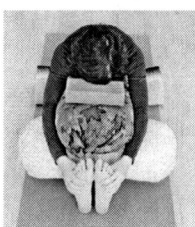

Supported Paschimottanasana
(page 76)
1 to 4 minutes

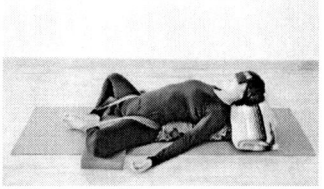

Supta Baddha Konasana
(page 97)
15 to 30 minutes

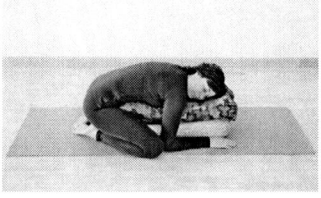

Supported Balasana
(page 71)
5 to 10 minutes

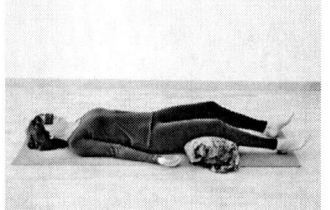

Savasana
(page 117)
10 to 20 minutes

Finish in seated meditation with Pranayama:

Ujjayi
(page 56)
1 minute

Nadi Shodana
(page 57)
3-5 minutes

Sequence for Pregnancy

A general focus on connecting with your baby, resting your body and nourishing yourself can be taken while practicing this sequence.

Warm-up Series (page 32) 10-20 minutes

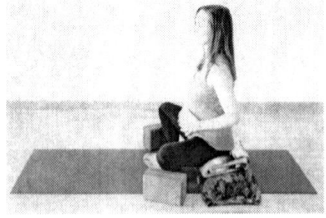

Supported Baddha Konasana

(page 123)

15 seconds to 2 minutes

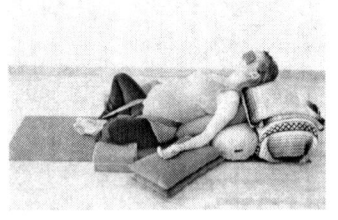

Elevated Supta Baddha Konasana

(page 143)

5 to 20 minutes

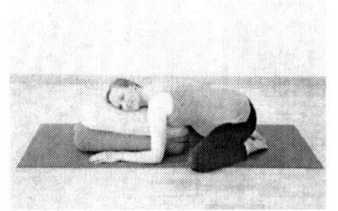

Modified Supported Balasana

(page 131)

2 to 10 minutes

(1 to 5 minutes with head to each side)

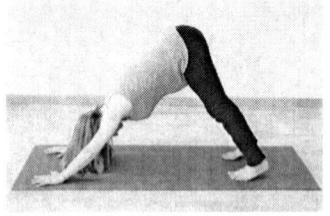

Adho Mukha Svanasana

(page 137)

15 seconds to 1 minute

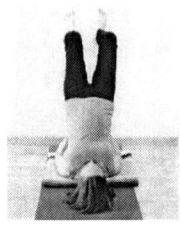

Salamba Sarvangasana, with wall

(page 140)

10 seconds to 5 minutes

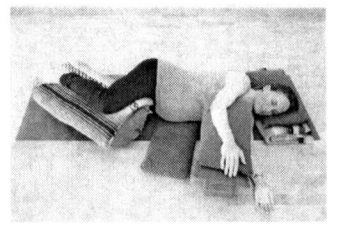

Side-Lying Savasana

(page 151)

5 to 20 minutes

Sequence for Postnatal 1

Just after Birth (1 day to 2 months, longer if needed). After your baby is born is another time when a restorative practice can help tremendously in recuperating from the birth and helping to adjust and to ease some of the stress that can come with this next chapter in your life. Any one of these poses can be practiced on their own if you are limited with time.

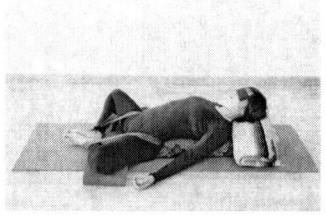

Supta Baddha Konasana
(page 97)
10 to 20 minutes

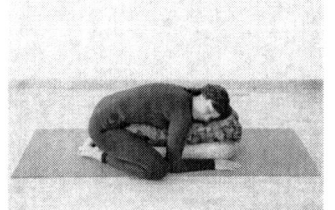

Supported Balasana
(page 71)
5 to 10 minutes

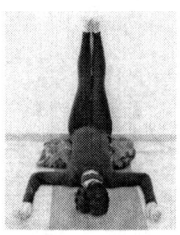

Viparita Karani
(page 89)
5 to 15 minutes

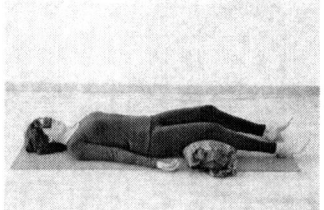

Savasana
(page 117)
10 to 20 minutes

Sequence for Postnatal 2

After the sixth week with a vaginal birth and the tenth week with a cesarean a more active yoga practice can be taken. The restorative practice can be expanded and continue being practiced.

Warm-up Series (page 32)

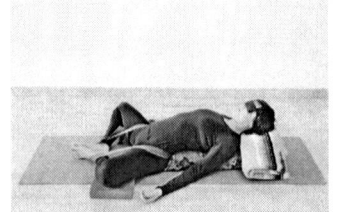

Supta Baddha Konasana
(page 97)
5 to 20 minutes

Ujjayi (page 56) 1 minute

Nadi Shodana (page 57)
3 to 5 minutes

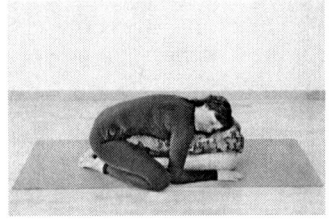

Supported Balasana
(page 71)
5 to 7 minutes

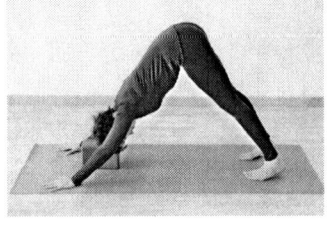

Adho Mukha Svanasana
(page 79)
30 seconds to 2 minutes

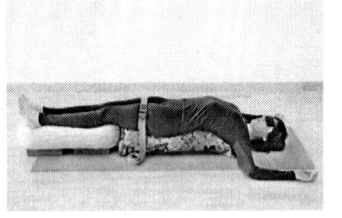

Setubandha Sarvangasana
(page 82)
1 to 10 minutes

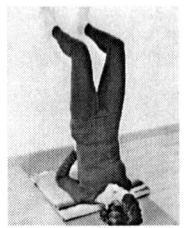

Salamba Sarvangasana,
with wall support
(page 93)
30 seconds to 5 minutes

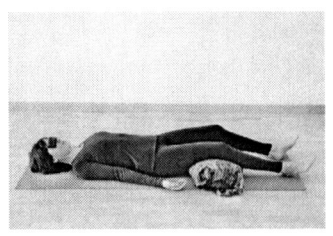

Savasana,
with knees on bolster
(page 117)
5 to 30 minutes

Sequencing

A General Sequence for Stress, Anxiety, Fibromyalgia or Chronic Fatigue

Warm-up Series (page 32)
Tadasana (Mountain Pose)

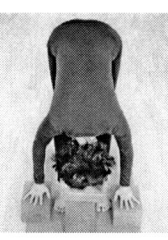 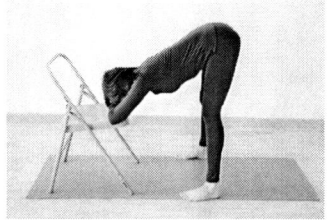

Standing Supported Uttanasana
(page 66)
1 to 5 minutes

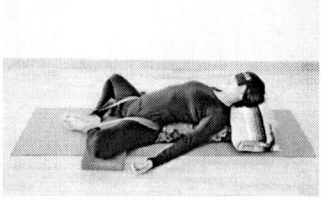

Supta Baddha Konasana
(page 97)
10 to 30 minute

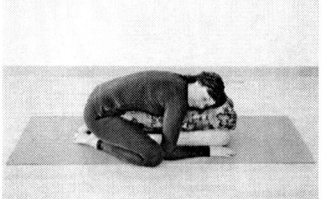

Supported Balasana
(page 71)
3 to 10 minutes

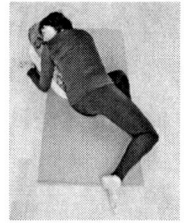

Supported Balasana, twisting variation
(page 114)
30 seconds to 2 minutes each side

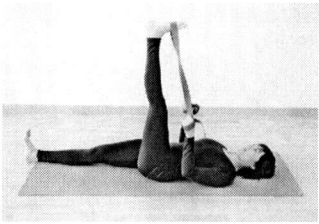 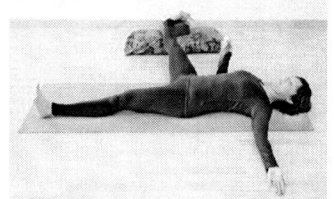 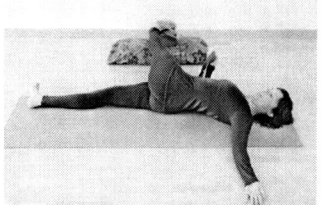

Supta Padangusthasana
(page 107)
1 to 3 minutes per variation

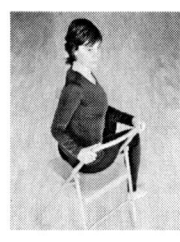 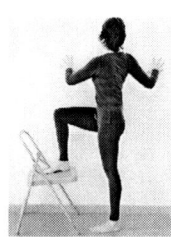

Marichyasana
seated and standing variation
(page 111)
30 seconds each side each variation

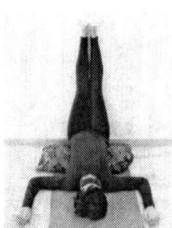 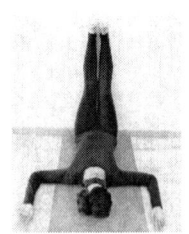

Viparita Karni

(page 89)

5 to 20 minutes

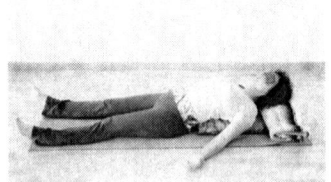

Supported Savasana,

with Ujjayi pranayama

(page 117, 56)

2 to 5 minutes

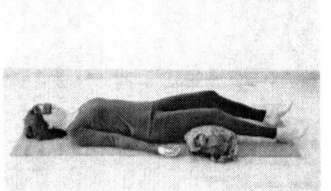

Savasana

(page 117)

10 to 25 minutes

Seated Nadi Shodana

(page 57)

3 to 10 minutes

Sequence for Depression (long)

Warm-up Series (page 32)
Tadasana (Mountain Pose)

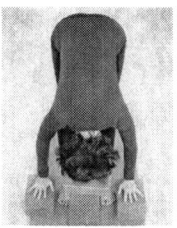
Uttanasana
with hand and head
support
(page 66)
1 to 5 minutes

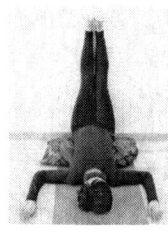
Viparita Karni
(page 89)
5 to 10 minutes

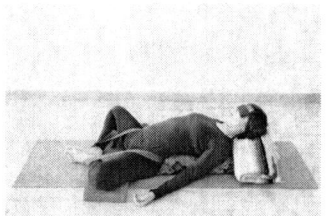
Supta Baddha Konasana
(page 97)
10 to 20 minutes

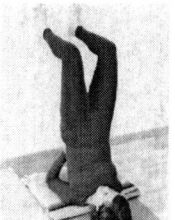
Salamba Sarvangasana
with wall support
(page 93)
2 to 5 minutes

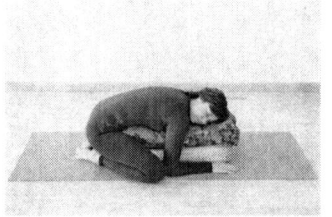
Supported Balasana
(page 71)
3 to 10 minutes

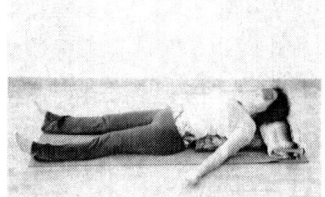
Supported Savasana
with Ujjayi pranayama
(page 117, 56)
2 to 5 minutes

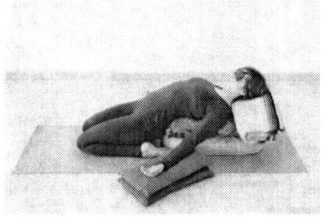
Supta Virasana
(page 103)
30 seconds to
10 minutes

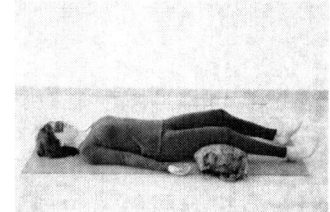
Savasana
(page 117)
10 to 25 minutes

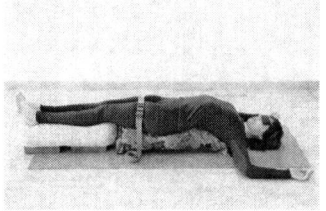
**Setubandha
Sarvangasana**
(page 82)
5 to 15 minutes

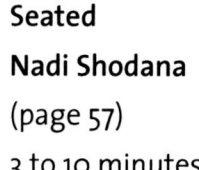
**Seated
Nadi Shodana**
(page 57)
3 to 10 minutes

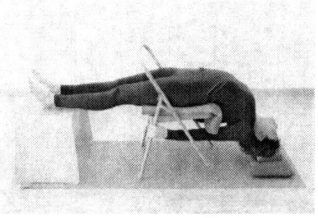
Viparita Dandasana
(page 86)
15 seconds to 5 minutes

Sequence for Depression (short)

Warm-up Series (page 32)
Tadasana (Mountain Pose)

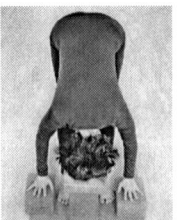
Uttanasana
with hand and head
support
(page 66)
1 to 4 minutes

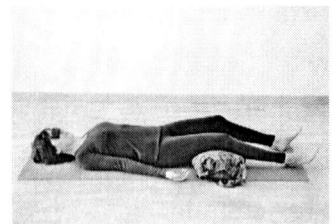
Savasana
(page 117)
10 to 25 minutes

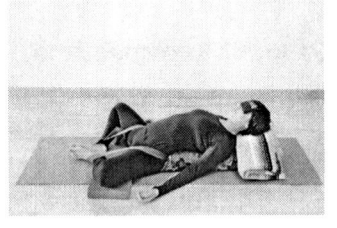
Supta Baddha Konasana
(page 97)
10 to 20 minutes

**Seated
Nadi Shodana**
(page 57)
1 to 5 minutes

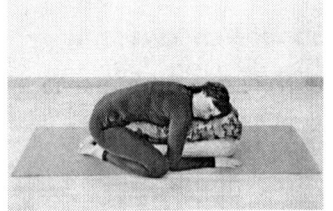
Supported Balasana
(page 71)
3 to 10 minutes

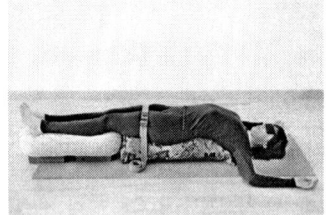
**Setubandha
Sarvangasana**
(page 82)
5 to 15 minutes

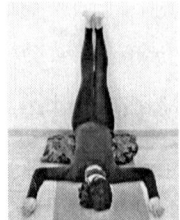
Viparita Karni
(page 89)
5 to 10 minutes

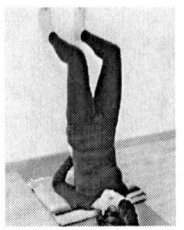
Salamba Sarvangasana
with wall support
(page 93)
30 seconds to 5 minutes

Sequence for Depression (shorter)

Warm-up Series (page 32)
Tadasana (Mountain Pose)

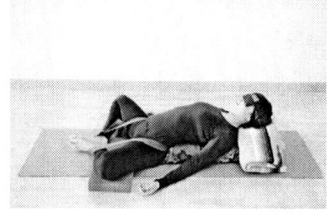

Supta Baddha Konasana
(page 97)
10 to 20 minutes

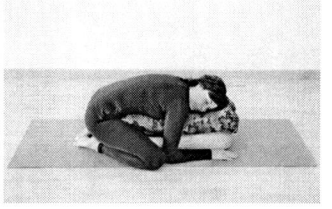

Supported Balasana
(page 71)
3 to 5 minutes

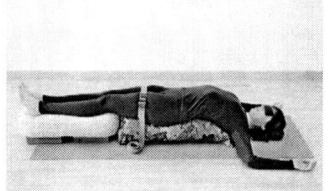

Setubandha Sarvangasana
(page 82)
2 to 10 minutes

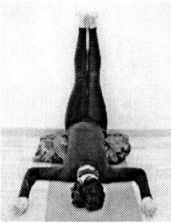

Viparita Karni
(page 89)
2 to 10 minutes

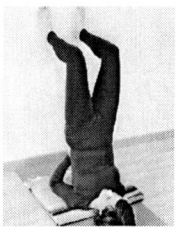

Salamba Sarvangasana
with wall support
(page 93)
30 seconds to 5 minutes

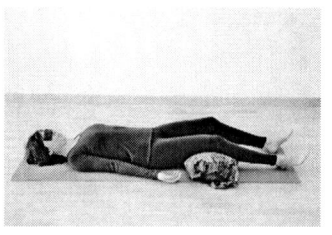

Savasana
(page 117)
10 to 20 minutes

Sequence for Exhaustion

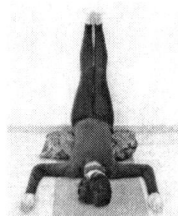
Viparita Karni
flat or elevated
(page 89)
5 to 10 minutes

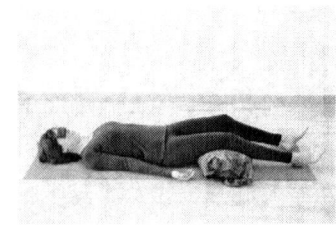
Savasana
with legs on bolster
(page 117)
10 to 20 minutes

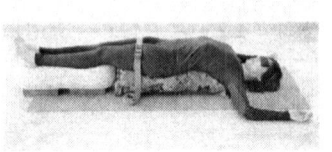
Supported Setubandha Sarvangasana
(page 82)
5 to 10 minutes

Seated Nadi Shodana
(page 57)
3 to 10 minutes

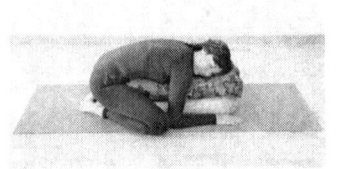
Supported Balasana
(page 71)
5 to 10 minutes

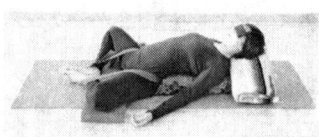
Supta Baddha Konasana
(page 97)
10 to 20 minutes

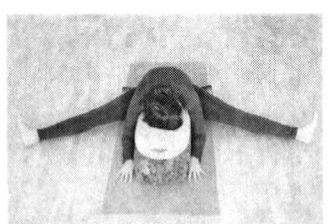
Supported Upavista Konasana
(page 68)
2 to 5 minutes

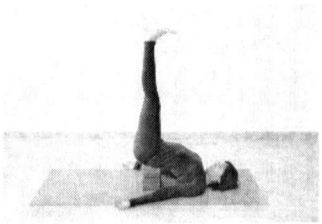
Salamba Sarvangasana
on wall, chair or block
(page 93)
3 to 5 minutes

Sequence for Headache

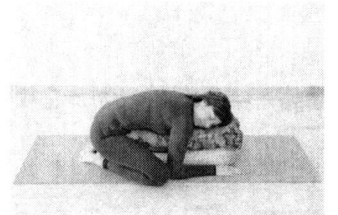
Supported Balasana
(page 71)
5 to 10 minutes

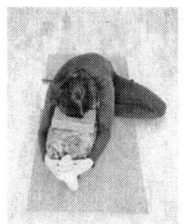
Supported Janu Sirsasana
(page 74)
1 to 5 minutes

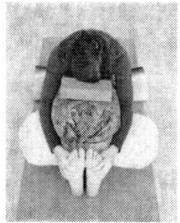
Supported Paschimottanasana
(page 76)
1 to 5 minutes

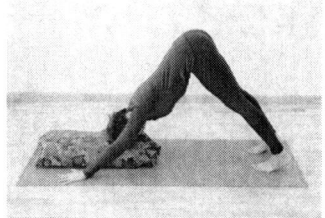
Adho Mukha Svanasana
(page 79)
30 seconds to 2 minutes

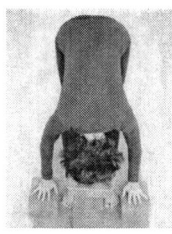
Standing Supported Uttanasana
(page 66)
1 to 5 minutes

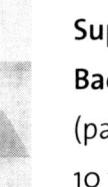
Supported Supta Baddha Konasana
(page 97)
10 to 20 minutes

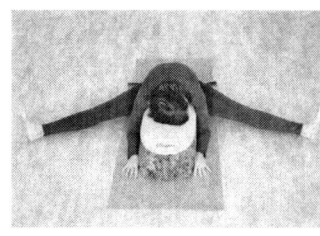
Supported Upavista Konasana
(page 68)
1 to 5 minutes

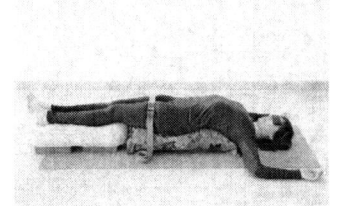
Supported Setubandha Sarvangasana
(page 82)
3 to 15 minutes

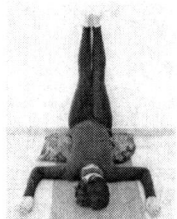
Viparita Karni
(page 89)
5 to 15 minutes

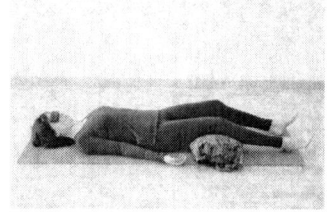
Savasana
(page 117)
10 to 20 minutes

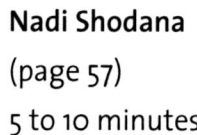
Nadi Shodana
(page 57)
5 to 10 minutes

Sequence for PMS

(Modified from *Yoga, The Path to Holistic Health*, B.K.S. Iyengar, pages 360-361)

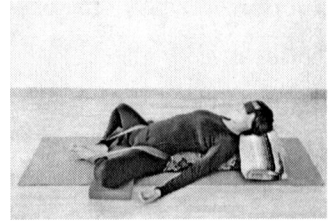

Supta Baddha Konasana
(page 97)
5 to 15 minutes

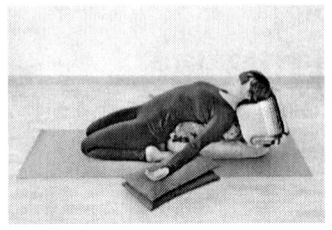

Supta Virasana
(page 103)
30 seconds to 5 minutes

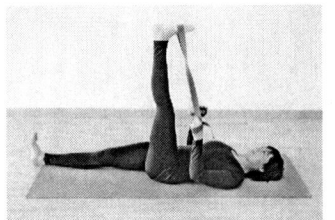 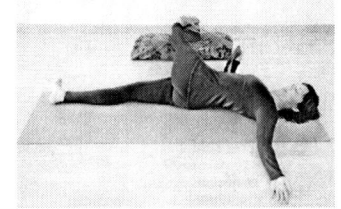

Supta Padangusthasana
(page 107)
2 to 4 minutes
each variation

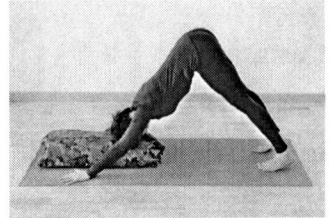

Adho Mukha Svanasana
(page 79)
30 seconds to 2 minutes

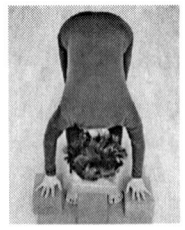

Uttanasana
(page 66)
1 to 5 minutes

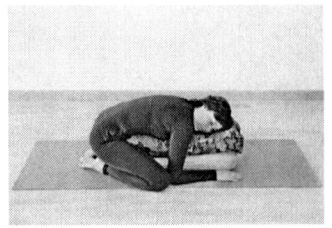

Supported Balasana
(page 71)
5 to 10 minutes

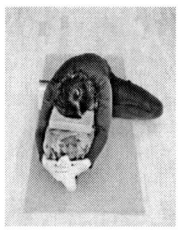

Janu Sirsasasana
(page 74)
2 to 5 minutes

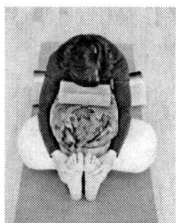

Paschimottanasana
(page 76)
2 to 5 minutes

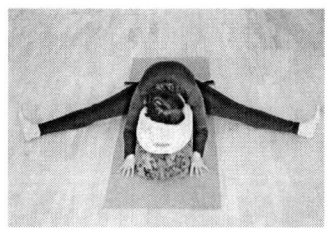

Upavista Konasana
(page 68)
2 to 5 minutes

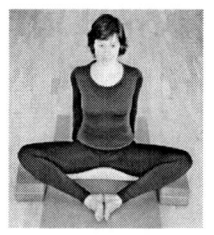

Baddha Konasana
(page 63)
30 seconds to 2 minutes

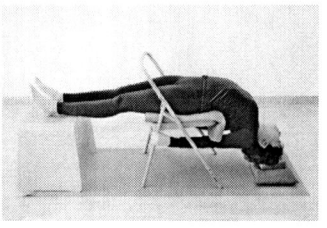

Viparita Dandasana
(page 86)
15 seconds to 5 minutes

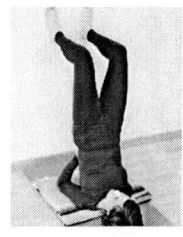

Salamba Sarvangasana
(page 93)
30 seconds to 10 minutes

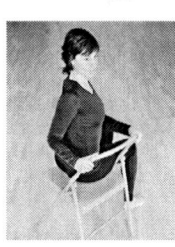 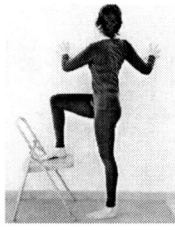

Utthita Marichyasana
(page 111)
30 seconds to 1 minutes each side, both variations

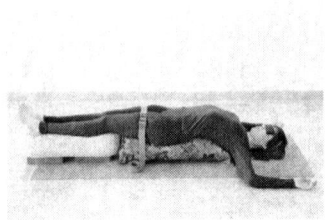

Setubandha Sarvangasana

(page 82)

2 to 15 minutes

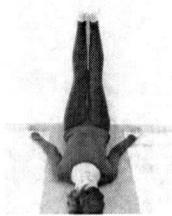

Viparita Karni

(page 89)

5 to 15 minutes

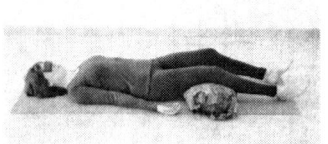

Savasana

(page 117)

5 to 30 minutes

Ujjayi

(page 56)

1 minute

Nadi Shodana

(page 57)

1 to 5 minutes

Sequence for Menstruation

(Modified from *Yoga, the Path to Holistic Health*, B.K.S. Iyengar, pages 356 - 358)

Warm-up Series (page 32), 10 to 30 minutes

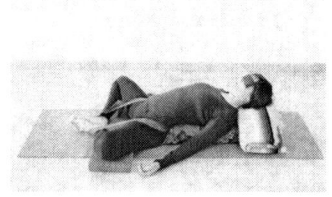
Supta Baddha Konasana
(page 97)
5 to 15 minutes

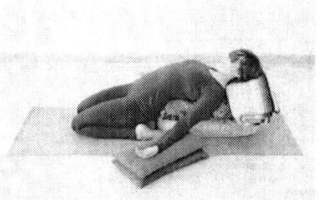
Supta Virasana
(page 103)
30 seconds to 5 minutes

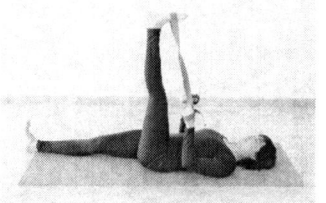 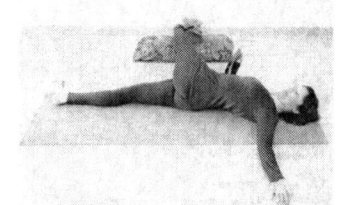
Supta Padangusthasana
(page 107)
2 to 5 minutes
each variation

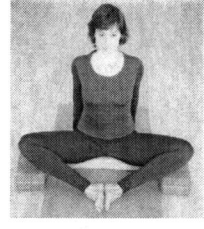
Baddha Konasana
(page 63)
1 to 3 minutes

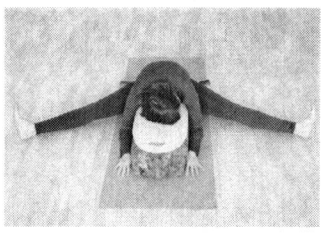
Upavista Konasana
(page 68)
2 to 5 minutes

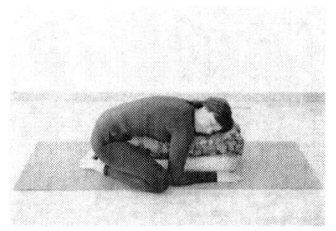
Supported Balasana
(page 71)
5 to 10 minutes

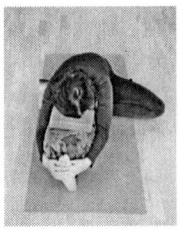
Janu Sirsasana
(page 74)
2 to 5 minutes per side

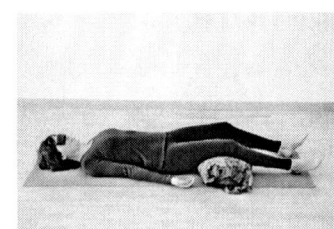
Savasana
(page 114)
5 to 25 minutes

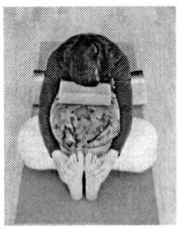
Pachimottanasana
(page 76)
2 to 5 minutes

Ujjayi
(page 54)
1 to 3 minutes

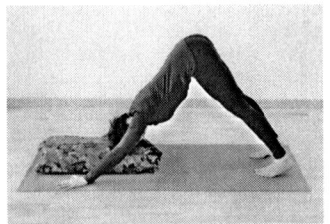
Adho Mukha Svanasana
(page 79)
30 seconds to 2 minutes

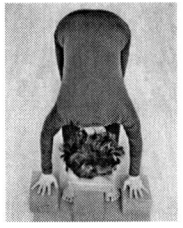
Uttanasana
(page 66)
1 to 5 minutes

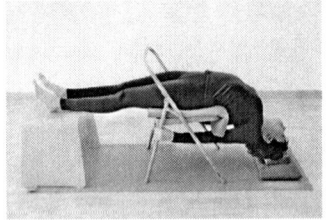
Viparita Dandasana
(page 86)
15 seconds to 3 minutes

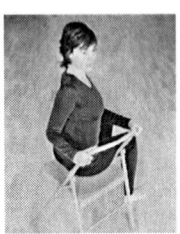
Utthita Marichyasana
(page 111)
30 seconds to 4 minutes (15 sec. to 2 min. per side)

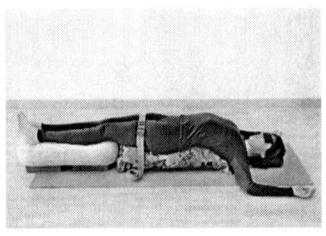
Setubandha Sarvangasana
(page 82)
10 to 20 minutes

Sequence for Menopause

(Modified from *Yoga, the Path to Holistic Health*, B.K.S. Iyengar, pages 361 - 364)

Warm-up Series (page 30), 10 to 30 minutes

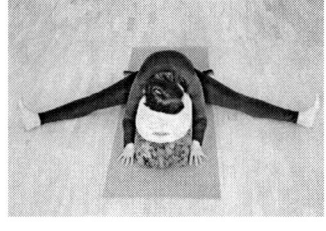

Upavista Konasana
(page 68)
2 to 5 minutes

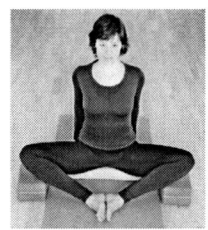

Baddha Konasana
(page 63)
1 to 3 minutes

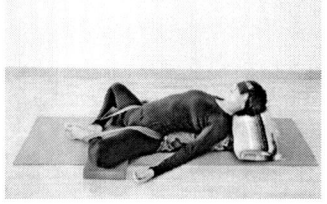

Supta Baddha Konasana
(page 97)
15 to 25 minutes

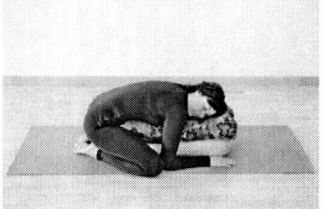

Supported Balasana
(page 71)
2 to 10 minutes

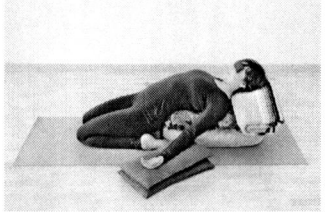

Supta Virasana
(page 103)
30 seconds to 5 minutes

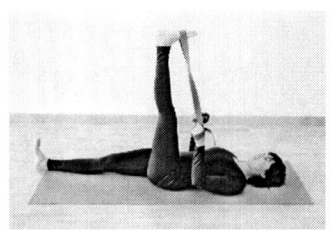 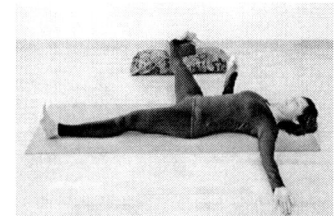 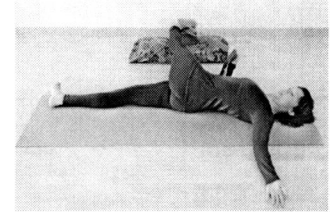

Supta Padangusthasana
(page 107)
1 to 4 minutes
each variation

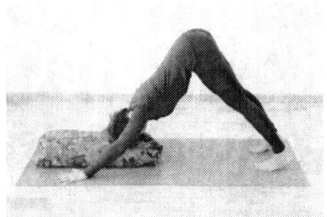

Adho Mukha Svanasana

(page 79)

30 seconds to 2 minutes

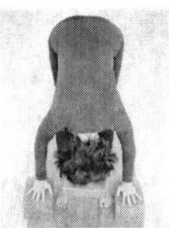

Uttanasana

(page 66)

30 seconds to 5 minutes

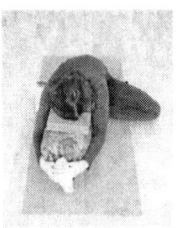

Janu Sirsasana

(page 74)

1 to 4 minutes per side

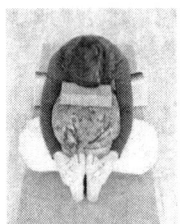

Pachimottanasana

(page 76)

1 to 5 minutes

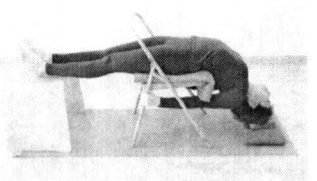

Viparita Dandasana

(page 86)

30 seconds to 3 minutes

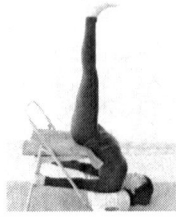

Salamba Sarvangasana

(page 93)

30 seconds to 5 minutes

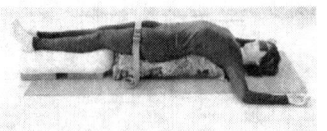

Setubandha Sarvangasana

(page 82)

1 to 10 minutes

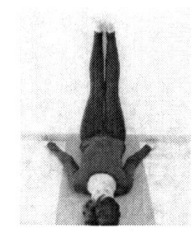 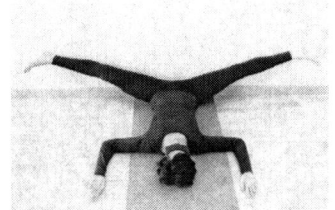 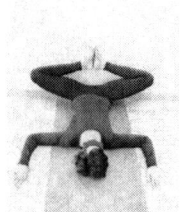

Viparita Karni
(page 89)
5 to 10 minutes

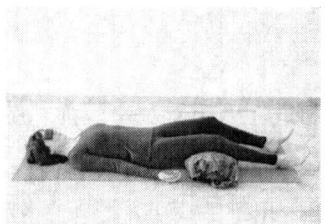

Savasana
(page 117)
10 to 25 minutes

Ujjayi
(page 56)
30 seconds to 3 minutes

Nadi Shadona
(page 57)
1 to 10 minutes

About the Author

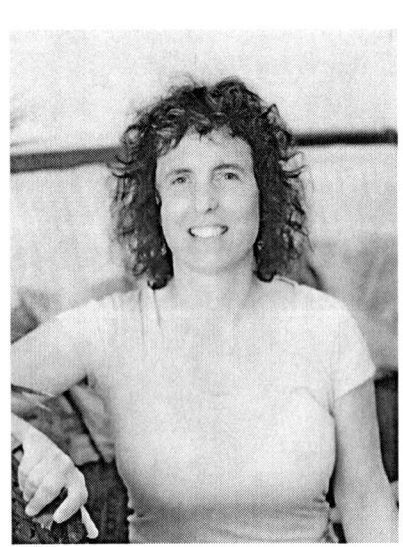

Puja Sue Flamm (Susana), 500 RYT, International Yoga Teacher, Yoga Teacher Trainer, Certified Massage Therapist, has been teaching yoga for almost 30 years. She has led numerous retreats, workshops and thousands of classes in the USA, China, Guatemala, Mexico, Cuba and Spain. Sue took her first meditation class in Transcendental Meditation at age 12, her first Hatha Yoga class at age 16 and has continued her study and practice throughout her rich and diverse life. She lived for six years at Kripalu Center where she was on staff as a yoga teacher, massage therapist, program director and cook. She has co-owned two yoga centers, and ran an education center for pre- and postnatal education and yoga. Originally certified in Kripalu Yoga, she went on to study Iyengar, Ashtanga and Anusara yoga styles. Sue draws from a wealth of teaching experience and personal practices. Devoted to her students and to the teachings of the eight-fold path of yoga and Buddhism, she is continually deepening her understanding of yoga, Buddhist philosophy and meditation. She uses yoga, Buddhist meditation techniques, visualizations, informed hands-on assists and her compassionate loving presence to guide her students to a deeper connection with the body, physical alignment, understanding of the mind and connecting to spirit. Her teaching encourages physical opening, strengthening of the muscular and organ systems, bridging interconnections within, deep relaxation and the cultivation of loving kindness.

For more information about Sue and her teaching schedule, check the pujayoga.net website.

About the Models

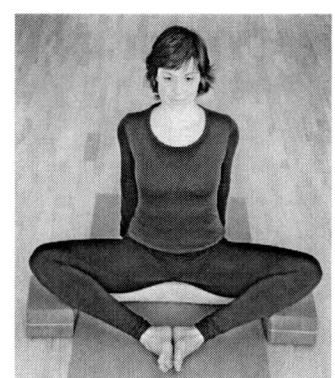

Jennifer Susan Kaiser has been a yogini since four years old when she was entranced by Lilias Folan, whom she watched regularly. Jenny was born in Oakland, California; her work today among other things is as an eclectic personal trainer and somatic movement educator. A certified massage therapist from Baltimore School of Massage and a certified Yamuna Bodyrolling instructor, her yogic style influences are Body Mind Centering and Donna Farhi. She lives in Valencia, Spain, and loves going for long international motorcycle trips with her favorite playmate and movement inspiration, her husband.

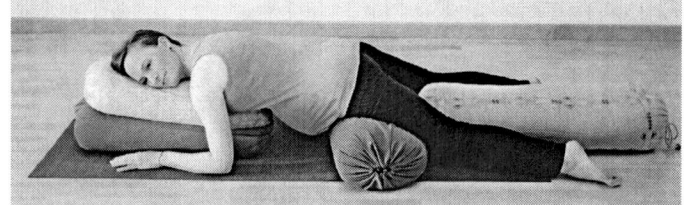

Julia was introduced to practicing yoga from an early age, spending large parts of her childhood in Ibiza, Spain. She intensified her practice at the Life Centre in Nottinghill, London, which she frequented for seven years. Since living in Valencia she has attended prenatal classes with Carmela Escriche and practiced postnatal yoga with Susana Flamm. Julia is expecting her second daughter.

The Photographer

Pablo Latorre Garcia is an international photographer. He was born in Valencia, Spain in 1978.

References

These books were useful references as I was writing and in my years of teaching. I recommend them for anyone looking for further reading.

- *Rest and Renew* by Judith Lasater, Ph.D
- *Yoga, the Path to Holistic Health* by B.K.S. Iyengar
- *The Blooming of a Lotus* by Thich Nhat Hanh
- *Back Care Basics* by Mary Pullig Schatz, MD
- *Healing Mantras* by Tomas Ashley-Farrand
- *The Hidden Messages in Water* by Dr. Masaru Emoto
- *Loving What Is* by Byron Katie
- *The Relaxation Response* by Miriam Z. Klipper and Herbert Benson

The following references were also helpful, particularly for the specific chapters they're mentioned in.

Chapter 1

T.K.V. Desikachar, *The Heart of Yoga* (Inner Traditions International, 1999).
M. Govindan, *Babaji and the 18 Siddha Kriya Yoga Tradition* (Kriya Yoga Publications, 1991).
B.K.S. Iyengar, *Light on Yoga* (Random House, 1995 and Schocken Books, 1995).
Barbara Stoler Miller (trans.), *Yoga: Discipline of Freedom: The Yoga Sutras Attributed to Patanjali* (Bantam Books, 1998).
Alberto Villoldo, *Yoga, Power and Spirit: Patanjali the Shaman* (Hay House, 2007).
Cynthia Worby, *The Everything Yoga Book* (Adams Media, 2002).

http://www.self-realization.com/articles/yoga/yoga_systems.htm
http://www.sivananda.org/teachings/fourpaths.html#jnana
http://www.swamij.com/history-yoga.htm

Chapter 7

Thich Nhat Hanh, *The Miracle of Mindfulness: An Introduction to the Practice of Meditation* (Beacon Press, 1999).
Esther M. Sternberg, *The Balance Within: The Science Connecting Health & Emotions* (W.H. Freeman & Co., 2000; paperback: Times Books/Henry Holt, 2001).

Esther M. Sternberg, http://blip.tv/slowtv/emotions-the-brain-and-the-body-p1-esther-sternberg-and-ian-hickie-4414940.

Shawn Talbott, *The Cortisol Connection* (2nd edn., Hunter House, 2007).

Shelley E. Taylor, "Tend and befriend: Biobehavioral bases of affiliation under stress" (2006) Current Directions in Psychological Science 15(6); http://taylorlab.psych.ucla.edu/2006_Tend%20and%20Befriend_Biobehavioral%20Bases%20of%20Affiliation%20Under%20Stress.pdf.

Constantine Tsigos, George P. Chrousos, "Hypothalamic–pituitary–adrenal axis, neuroendocrine factors and stress" (2002) Journal of Psychosomatic Research 53:865–871.

http://theweek.com/article/index/209353/stress-in-america-5-unnerving-new-facts (November 2010).

Chapters 10, 11 and 12

The main resources used for translations, posture benefits, contraindications and to provide parts of some of the sequencing were:

B.K.S. Iyengar, *Yoga, The Path to Holistic Health*; Judith Lasater, *Rest and Renew*; and www.YogaJournal.com.

Further References

J. Carmody et al., "A pilot study of mindfulness-based stress reduction for hot flashes" (2006) Menopause 13(5):760-769.

P.J. Mansky & D.B. Wallerstedt, "Complementary medicine in palliative care and cancer symptom management" (2006) Cancer Journal 12(5):425-431.

Todd Neale, "PTSD relief comes with a mantra" (June 03, 2011) MedPage Today.

Robert Nilsson, Pictures of the brain's activity during Yoga Nidra, http://www.yogameditation.com/Articles/Issues-of-Bindu/Bindu-11/Pictures-of-the-brain-s-activity-during-Yoga-Nidra.

"Reiki Really Works: A Groundbreaking Scientific Study" http://greenlotus.hubpages.com/hub/Reiki_Really_Works-A_Groundbreaking_Scientific_Study.

Susan Seligson, "Your brain on yoga: Calmer, more content; MED study: Mood benefits edge out those of walking" (2011) Commonwealth; http://www.bu.edu/bostonia/winter-spring11/yoga/.

R.S. Surwit et al., "Stress management improves long-term glycemic control in type 2 diabetes" (2002) Diabetes Care 25:30-34.